# CHOOSE YOUR FOODS

## like your life depends on them

To my patients

# CHOOSE YOUR FOODS

## like your life depends on them


Naturopathic Medical Doctor

Foreword by
New York Times best-selling author
Dr. Joseph Mercola

Including the popular articles from the www.mercola.com website:

"How to Cook Whole Foods from Scratch
and Keep Your Day Job,"

"How to Raise a Whole Food Child
in a Processed Food World,"

"The Sweet Tooth: Defeating the Little Rascal"

and

"If you crave this . . . what you really want and need is . . . "

COLLEEN HUBER
NATUROPATHIC MEDICAL DOCTOR

**Previous editions copyrighted 2007, 2008.**

ISBN: Softcover 978-0-692-39888-3



This book was printed in the United States of America.

Medical Choice Editions

# Foreword

## by Dr. Joseph Mercola

Optimizing your diet is an essential tool to better health as Naturopathic Physician Colleen Huber's book so effectively illustrates. Dr. Huber has contributed some outstanding articles to www.Mercola.com, the most visited natural health website, with approximately 3 million viewers per month.

Dr. Huber's strong ability to communicate will help you with practical and convenient ways to work healthy eating habits and wholesome food into your daily schedule. Sadly, our focus on technology, innovation and knowledge and time pressures make it very easy to resort to processed and convenience foods.

She helps guide your personal health journey by looking toward a future of improved eating habits that will help orient you to implementing the changes that will provide you with positive health benefits. Her coaching helps you avoid feelings of guilt

and dependence regarding previous food choices that shackle your mind and keep you stuck in crave-and-binge cycles. Rewire your mind and your kitchen for healthier choices that eliminate physical cravings and allow you to achieve the enjoyable state of health that you desire. Dr. Huber shows you just how feasible it really is to eat whole organic foods. Although organic food has a reputation for being outrageously expensive, and, indeed, it has much room for improvement price-wise, there are many times when it is actually less expensive than commercially prepared food if you just check labels and sales.

She explains why the philosophy of eating everything in moderation may not be the best choice for you. While it's certainly a good idea to eat a varied diet, that variety shouldn't include highly processed foods or other low-quality food items (like farm-raised fish, pasteurized milk and soda) because contrary to what you might think, even a little bit can hurt you.

The other major problem with eating 'everything in moderation' has to do with your metabolic type. Even healthy foods like vegetables can be fine-tuned for your specific type, and depending on whether you're a protein type, a carb type or a mixed type, certain vegetables (or meats, nuts, fruits, etc.) will be healthier for you than others. That said, 'everything in moderation' can be a good motto, but only if you limit 'everything' to healthy foods that balance your metabolic type. If you'd like to find out your own metabolic type, see my website, www.Mercola.com and type "metabolic type" in the search bar.

Eliminating sugar from your diet is critical to optimizing health, as the chapters on The Sweet Tooth well describe. Along with sugar, grains pose a challenge and often unidentified risk. Most grains break down to sugar very rapidly and can cause the same problems with insulin dysregulation.

As a clinician, one of the most challenging tasks I face is offering simple practical guidelines that allow a parent to implement the diet recommendations that I know will turn their child's health around. As a mother who has gone through this drill on multiple occasions, Dr. Huber draws from her real world experience to fill this gap with her chapters on children's food, which provide a marvelous tool for parents to implement.

Her parenting skills also assist her in describing the diligent work it takes to raise a young child in a healthy environment among many temptations and distractions. About the only area Dr. Huber didn't cover in her comprehensive chapters on children's health is an important one when you're transitioning your child into better health habits: Get them moving away from the couch to the playground. In fact, running or jumping – instead of swimming and biking may be the best way for your kids to strengthen their bones.

Many parents are filled with fear about fevers in their children. Dr. Huber helps you understand that supporting your child's fever instead of immediately going to the medicine cabinet for a fever-reducing acetaminophen is one of the best things you can do for your child's fever. She has a comprehensive section on the benefits of fever and why supporting a fever is an effective form of treatment.

It is common knowledge that it is far easier to prevent an illness than to treat it. This involves building up and keeping the immune system functioning strong before an illness gets the chance to invade. Proper hygiene is critical to achieving and maintaining optimal health and just as Huber points out, it's the germs that require special attention. This can be a difficult area to monitor particularly with children as they are constantly engaged in some form of hand-to-mouth contact and germ

transmission, and Dr. Huber has a number of helpful suggestions in this area.

If you are looking for a basic book with sound advice on how to conveniently work healthy foods into your life, either for yourself alone or your family, then this book will take you there and provide a pleasant and fascinating read at the same time. Dr. Huber's practical guide will help you live a life full of vibrant energy that is free from the constant struggles of chronic health challenges.

Dr. Mercola
Founder of Mercola.com
World's most visited natural health site

# Contents

# About the Author

Colleen Huber, NMD is a Naturopathic Medical Doctor and a Naturopathic Oncologist (Fellow of the Naturopathic Oncology Research Institute, FNORI), licensed in Arizona, USA. She completed her medical training at Southwest College of Naturopathic Medicine in Tempe, AZ and Total Wellness Medical Center in 2006.

Dr. Huber is President of the Naturopathic Cancer Society. She owns a naturopathic cancer clinic in Tempe, AZ. Her website NatureWorksBest.com has the most comprehensive data of any cancer clinic, whether conventional or natural, on the results obtained from naturopathic treatments for cancer. She has written for the world's most visited health site, www.Mercola.com, on matters of nutrition and naturopathic medicine. Dr. Huber has been interviewed on television and radio throughout the U.S. Her article *"Glycemic restriction in cancer patients"* was published in Cancer Strategies Journal in April 2014. Dr. Huber was lead author of the study "*Cholesterol and diet in cancer survivors,*" presented to the International Congress of Naturopathic Medicine, July 2014.

# Introduction:
# Andrew Weil, MD demands that the medical profession learn nutrition

At a conference of health professionals in Tucson, Arizona, Andrew Weil, MD of the University of Arizona Integrative Medicine Program challenged conventional physicians with the following problems:

- Less than 6% of medical school graduates receive adequate training in clinical nutrition, according to the American Journal of Clinical Nutrition. Weil said, "The current state of nutrition education of health professionals is non-existent to substandard."
- More than 20% of hospitals have fast food restaurants on their premises.
- Obesity is quickly becoming the #1 cause of preventable death in the U.S.
- Some consequences of nutritional illiteracy among physicians are:

Physicians are unable to counsel patients about optimum diet or make use of dietary change as a primary therapeutic intervention or help patients be informed consumers of dietary supplements.

Unless it establishes its credibility, the medical profession is unable to act as a social and political force to counteract the commercial pressures that have led to the ubiquity of fast food restaurants, soft drinks and low-quality vending machines in public schools, hospitals and other public places.

**Medical Schools Seek Help with Natural Medicine**

A two-year study [1] conducted by the National Center for Complementary and Alternative Medicine and released in 2004 found that fully one-third of Americans over the age of 18 use natural medicine treatments in maintaining health and treating illness. These methods include a diverse list of modalities - acupuncture, chiropractic, herbal medicine, clinical nutrition, homeopathy and massage. When prayer was included, nearly 2 out of 3 Americans use some form of alternative medicine treatment in their health regimen.

After 30 years of steadily increasing public demand for a more natural and humane side to medicine, natural therapies have come to be so much in demand that the majority of medical schools in the U.S. now offer some form of instruction in nontraditional therapies. Schools including Harvard Medical College, Johns Hopkins and Thomas Jefferson University have centers for complementary and alternative medicine.

Increasingly, patients are giving up on the conventional medical system and choosing acupuncturists, chiropractors, naturopaths and other holistic-minded doctors for their health care needs.

---

[1] Common Dreams New Center. San Francisco Chronicle reprint "Americans Broaden Concepts of Medicine". May 28, 2004.

Of these, only licensed naturopathic physicians have medical school training in both pharmaceutical and natural treatments, and know how to combine them or switch from one to the other safely and effectively. Yet at present, there are only about 3,000 naturopathic physicians in the U.S., which is only one for every 100,000 people.

# Part I
# Beginning with childhood

# Chapter 1
# When to start your baby on solid food

The Year 2000 Health Goals for the United States, "Healthy People 2000," recommends that mothers nurse their infants for at least 6 months. At that 6-month point a process occurs known as *weaning*, which is from the Anglo-Saxon *wenian*, which literally means "to become accustomed to something different." [2] Such a process does not imply a cessation of breastfeeding, but rather the addition of other foods.

Where did 6 months come from? The consensus seems to be as follows: The American Academy of Pediatrics Committee on Nutrition has concluded that no nutritional benefit is gained from starting solid foods before the age of 4-6 months.[3] The World Health Organization (WHO), the Canadian Pediatric Society, the Paediatric Society of New Zealand, and similar

---

[2] Schmitz J, McNeish A. Development of structure and function of the gastrointestinal tract: relevance for weaning. In Ballabriga A, Rey J, editors. *Weaning: why, what and when?* Workshop Series, vol 11, New York, 1987, Vevey/Raven.

[3] Committee on Nutrition, American Academy of Pediatrics. On the feeding of supplemental foods to infants, *Pediatrics* 65:1178, 1980.

organizations in other countries have made similar statements.[4] [5] [6]. In fact, before six months the epithelial lining of the gut is not sufficiently developed to handle solid foods. Too early feeding of solid foods is a cause of leaky gut, allowing large molecules to get into the bloodstream and create the antibodies that characterize long-term food sensitivity.

Of equal importance, your baby starts reaching for the food on your plate about the age of 6 months. The AAP Committee on Nutrition further states, "By 5 to 6 months of age, the infant will be able to indicate a desire for food by opening his or her mouth and leaning forward, and to indicate disinterest or satiety by leaning back and turning away."[7]

Breastfeeding anthropologist Katherine Dettwyler identifies 6 months as the age at which most human cultures throughout history have introduced solid foods. Around this 6-month point, there are very good reasons for continuing to breastfeed and very good reasons for supplementing high quality solid foods as well. Dettwyler notes, "Nonhuman primates and children in traditional cultures worldwide normally experience several years of a transitional diet, with steadily increasing amounts of solid foods in addition to breast milk. The breast milk component of the diet continues to provide an excellent, uncontaminated source of

---

[4] Canadian Pediatric Society Nutrition Committee: Infant feeding: a statement. *Can J Public Health* 70-376. 1979

[5] Department of Health and Social Security: *Present Day Practice in Infant Feeding: Studies on Health and Social Subjects.* London, 1977.

[6] World Health Organization: *Joint WHO/UNICEF meeting on infant and young child feeding*. Geneva 1979. WHO.

[7] Committee on Nutrition, American Academy of Pediatrics: Supplemental foods for infants. In Barnes LA, editor: *Pediatric Nutrition Handbook,* Elk Grove Village, IL, 1993. American Academy of Pediatrics.

protein as well as of immunological factors, and may be the only food the child desires or can tolerate during illnesses."[8]

> "The newborn baby has only three demands. They are warmth in the arms of its mother, food from her breast, and security in the knowledge of her presence. Breastfeeding satisfies all three."
>
> Grantly Dick-Read

First, let's examine the benefits of continued breastfeeding. Two to four years of breastfeeding is typical for modern humans, as shown by cross-cultural evidence from around the world.[9] The reasons for continued breastfeeding are many. Breast milk not only continues to be nutritionally preferable to any other formula or food for the infant and toddler, but it is also vastly more useful than artificial infant feeding products in immunological, biochemical and cognitive benefits. As long as a child is ingesting breastmilk, it is protective against a wide range of illnesses and parasites. It is also important for mothers to understand the life-long health advantages to their child of breastfeeding and conversely, without breastfeeding, the increased rates of morbidity and mortality during childhood, higher rates of cancer and diabetes during adulthood and weaker cognitive development.

On the other hand, sooner or later solid foods will have to be introduced, and for the reasons given above, you may start to think about the types and quantities of such foods as your child approaches six months.

---

[8] Dettwyler K. "Natural age at weaning in humans as derived from the comparative nonhuman primate life history data." In Stuart-Macadam P, Dettwyler K. *Breastfeeding: Bio-cultural Perspectives*. New York, 1995.
[9] Ibid.

Breast milk supplies sufficient protein for the first 6 or 7 months of life. Afterward, the growing infant requires additional protein for adequate growth. Public health guidelines are approximately 14 grams per day for infants under one year old and 16 grams for those aged 1-4. Most of this protein may still be supplied by breast milk and the remainder supplemented with other foods.

Consider your baby's first foods among those that are soft or easily gummed by the child. Such early foods may include:

- mashed avocado
- yam or sweet potato
- cooked peas, lentils or beans of various kinds
- mashed banana or papaya

A few months later, as more teeth begin to erupt, and the GI tract epithelium begins to mature, a more varied diet will be tolerated (and maybe even demanded!) by your baby. At this point, consider adding:

- Cooked greens, finely chopped, such as kale, chard, collards, spinach
- Squashes, such as butternut, acorn and other winter squashes
- Mashed asparagus
- Eggs
- Nut butters; organic Valencia peanuts seem to be free of aflatoxin.
- Seaweeds that become soft on soaking, such as wakame or nori

Early in the second year, you may want to introduce some meats, although some parents introduce these during the first year.

Watch your child carefully as he or she eats meat, as it is the most frequently choked-on category of food. You may consider:

- Chicken, turkey or other poultry
- Fish (Remember, only Pacific salmon[10] is least contaminated to completely free of mercury and PCBs.)
- Mozzarella cheese or other cheese that can be made soft by heating. Such cheeses can be baked on a casserole of some of the above vegetables and meats.
- Pieces of fruit cut small, (but no whole grapes yet).

Water and breastmilk of course, and never fruit juices or other beverages, should be given as the child desires.

Watch your child closely with all solid eating experiences for two main reasons. One, the novice eater chokes more easily and frequently than the rest of us. But it is also the easiest time to observe any food sensitivities. Introduce one new food at a time, and wait a few days before introducing the next one. That way, any unusual symptoms, such as redness of ears or cheeks, nasal discharge, darker areas under the eyes or puffy eyes, unusual moodiness, gassiness, vomiting or diarrhea may be attributed to the newly introduced food. When the suspect food is noted, discontinue temporarily and try it again in several months with especially careful observation.

Please note that the above list does not include macaroni or other pasta, which is often given to babies. (Nor - heaven forbid - do we need to give children sweetened foods or drink of any kind.) Pasta, sweets and other refined carbohydrates offer nothing nutritionally to your child, but do wreak havoc with your child's gut, immune system, neurological, endocrine and even cardiovascular health. Sticking with preferably organic whole foods through your child's earliest years of eating will develop the

---

[10] http://www.mercola.com/2003/may/10/farmed_salmon.htm

healthy taste preferences that you will later yearn for if you do not follow this advice. If preparing whole organic food seems too daunting a task, please see the other chapters on this topic:

Cook whole food from scratch and keep your day job

Children's food demands: do you have to give in?

The Sweet Tooth: defeating the little rascal

# Chapter 2
# Children's food demands:
# Do you have to give in?

Which choice should a parent make at a child's birthday party?

a) forbid your child to have cake and ice cream
b) not take your child to any birthday parties
c) take healthy food to the party for your child
d) take enough healthy food for everyone
e) let your child eat what everybody else is eating

Growing up in a family where sugar was not eaten, I actually have strong opinions on this matter. My father was the strict disciplinarian who never allowed any sugar, and either kept us away from other kids' birthday parties in order to avoid the aggravation, or let us go, but made us sit out the cake and ice cream festivities. My mother, on the other hand, pitied us deprived children and urged that we be allowed some treats, if only for social mingling. Relatives fretted that we would not turn out normal. Friends stuck by us, but worried that other friends would reject us for being "health nuts". Our teachers didn't know what to make of us. One of the first books I read in first grade even claimed that ice cream was a healthy food, and it seemed that my peers considered it to be one of the basic food groups, all of which certainly steamed my father. What was a small child to believe?

Actually, as long as I can remember, I have always been grateful that my father's view prevailed over (or drowned out) all others, and that I have avoided any sugar cravings, sugar illness or withdrawal to this day. It may seem odd to read a term such as sugar illness, but I suspect the reason that I have never had headaches, PMS, depression, hypertension or weight gain, despite eating like a horse my whole life, has everything to do with not having sugar in my diet. Marrying late, my husband and I conceived our first child on our first attempt. I was 41 at the time. Is it a coincidence that I have never had sugar in my diet? Both sugar consumption and infertility are at all-time highs and worsening in recent decades.

But sugar illness goes far beyond the above-symptoms. Diabetes and obesity are epidemic in this country, and quickly increasing around the world. They, as well as cancer, feed directly on sugar. Cancer's fuel for growth is sugar.[11] [12] Hypertension due to arterial smooth muscle overgrowth and atherosclerosis have been tied in numerous studies to insulin in the bloodstream. Uffe Ravnskov, MD, a many-times awarded medical researcher, has shown through his study of the Masai people of Tanzania that they have the cleanest arteries in the world on their traditional diet of only meat, blood and milk (no sugar, no insulin). However, Masai who

---

[11] Fedirko V, et al. Glycemic index, glycemic load, dietary carbohydrate, and dietary fiber intake and risk of liver and biliary tract cancer in Western Europeans. Ann Oncol. 2013 Feb. 24(2). 543-553.
[12] Tavani A et al. Consumption of sweet foods and breast cancer risk in Italy. Ann Oncol. 2006 Feb. 17(2). 341-345.

migrate to cities with more westernized cuisine with refined carbs both in and out of Africa develop Western-type cardiovascular diseases. [13] [14]

In fact, insulin, rather than sugar itself may be the most serious problem. Studies of centenarians show almost nothing in common; some smoke, some don't; some are active, some aren't; some are serene, some are excitable. However, what they did have in common was low blood sugar and low insulin.[15] [16]

Now that I am a parent myself, I desperately want to pass on all the health advantages I have had over the years. My first inclination then is to confront anyone offering candy and the like. However, as a parent, I also try to find or create situations within social events in which my child does not have to feel unpleasantly isolated. So my choice on the multiple-choice question above is d) to provide enough alternative food for everybody at the party.

First, when I call to accept the invitation, I let the mom or dad know that we don't eat any sugar at all. If they are completely uncomprehending, I describe the problem as an allergy, which given all the pathology, it is. Then I offer to bring whole fruit, nuts, carrot, cucumber and celery sticks, cheese, watermelon-only popsicles, etc. for everyone.[17] Then while the cake is being cut, I

---

[13] Ravnskov, Uffe. The questionable role of saturated and polyunsaturated fatty acids in cardiovascular disease. J Clin Epidemiol. 1998 Jun; 51 (6).

[14] Ravnskov Uffe. Prevention of atherosclerosis in children. The Lancet. 2000; 355:69.

[15] Rosedale, Ron. Insulin and its metabolic effects. Presented at Designs for Health Institute's BoulderFest, August 1999 Seminar.

[16] Mercola, Joseph, Droege, Rachael. You should live to be at least 100. Find out how. www.mercola.com. 2003 Nov 15.

[17] Watermelon-only popsicles are the easiest recipe I know. Just stuff small chunks of watermelon fairly tightly into popsicle molds. Freeze for a whole fruit, unsweetened summer treat. Peach and plum also work.

distract my child with any interesting baby, pet or object handy. After the cake has been distributed, we then go get plates of whole food for ourselves and mingle freely. Older children, of course, are less appreciative of their parents' presence at a party, but are then old enough to be challenged with choosing only whole food for themselves, just as we expect them to refuse cigarettes and drugs. Also, after having been taught through their early childhood how their healthy, whole food diet can peacefully co-exist with their friends' different food choices, the older child and teenager can have the grace to maintain their friendships. This I know from personal experience. But there is another advantage these days that I could not enjoy as a teenager. Now that "Paleo" and "low carb" diets have become widely accepted, the whole food teen can stay popular with others just for being fashionable.

If your children demand poor quality food, it is because it has previously found its way into their school or your house, or has been advertised persuasively to them. If you demand more healthy whole food at your children's school, you won't be alone. Over two thirds of Arizona parents surveyed favored eliminating junk food machines from their children's schools. This was even after they were reminded in the survey that such machines were a source of income for cash-strapped schools.[18] Likewise, Waldorf schools often advertise an organic whole-food menu for the children.

If the food in your house is part of the problem, start shopping just the periphery of the supermarket where the whole foods are. Skip the aisles of processed and sweetened foods and drinks. Leaving bad food behind at the supermarket makes a whole food/sugar-free diet a whole lot easier. Whatever you do, don't bring the cookies and ice cream home to your kitchen, where they then sit there a few feet away from you like ticking bombs, and quickly find their way into everybody's tummies. (You are only

[18] Anne Ryman. Schools get big bucks in soda deals. The Arizona Republic. 2004 Jan 4.

human after all. Don't make your temptations any more difficult than they already are by bringing them into your house.) Start the clean sweep of your pantry during a summer break or long weekend, so that neither you nor your children will be tempted by junk outside the home within those first critical 48 hours. When the cravings become bothersome, massage all of both ears to cover the ear acupuncture points related to addiction. Broccoli, cheese and liver are foods high in chromium, which is helpful specifically for sugar cravings. Drinking water is the best way to flush out toxins and metabolites more quickly.

On creating a whole food household for the first time, your children may balk, but within a few days, they will 1) learn to accept the food that you are providing them, and 2) will then let you know that they are feeling better. You may be surprised at how well they can rise to the challenge. Children diagnosed with depression, when advised that if they stop eating sugar their depression will go away, usually rise to this challenge and heal themselves naturally without drugs. Grant your children this learning experience, and let them grow to be as grateful to you as I am to my wise father.

# Chapter 3
# Raising a whole food child in a processed food world

During at least some of childhood the grass is definitely greener elsewhere. One of the biggest challenges to your family's healthy lifestyle is your children's perception that other people are privileged simply because they eat differently. The parents' strategic awareness and preparation for the child's fascination with the Standard American Diet (SAD) is paramount.

Adults also fall into conforming to SAD just because so many other people are doing it. To which I respond: what law states that you must conform 100% to all majority cultural practices, including some of those practices that are kind of dumb?

At no time is the parents' advantage greater than in earliest childhood for understanding the crucial role of food in setting the course for either chronic disease or a lifetime of good health. At no other time is the parent's advantage greater for establishing a healthy routine. By the time the child is ready to start school, he or she is already developing a strong interest in being like their friends and doing what their friends are doing.

Use your advantage of a head start. You care way more about the quality of your child's food for several years, including pregnancy, before your child begins to feel pulled by the influence of those outside the family. Use that time to create a bubble of a near-perfectly healthy lifestyle that your child will get used to and will associate with home and family for the rest of his or her life. Changing to a whole food diet can of course be accomplished later, at the expense of tantrums, grumbling and other exaggerations of angst. The earlier you do it the easier.

An easy, healthy routine is your greatest strength, because when you start getting used to buying, preparing and eating whole organic foods, and when you make such foods the first thing that you reach for and the first impulse for meal preparation, then you are teaching your children their basic foundation diet and fulfilling their expectations of healthy good food being a part of their daily lives.

If you don't yet believe that whole food is easy, see the chapter, "Cook whole food from scratch and keep your day job." It will become second nature for them as well to reach for whole rather than processed foods, to value those produced without synthetic fertilizers, pesticides, MSG, sweeteners and preservatives. They learn from familiar experience to appreciate the great energized feeling that they get from a glass of raw milk or a handful of carrot sticks or a meal with dark leafy greens. If you are just now transitioning to a whole food diet, let your children fill up on as much whole healthy food as they want. The practical advantage of eating whole fresh foods is that they substitute, by their sheer bulk, the chemicals and denatured food derivatives that we might otherwise eat.

My suggestions for starting your kids off right are as follows:

1. The earlier you start the easier and the more effective your efforts. Breastfed kids have huge lifetime health advantages over formula fed babies. You will never again have the opportunity to make such a strong health impact in such a short amount of time, and for less effort and expense than formula feeding. Even if circumstances only allowed you to breastfeed your child for a short time, the advantages are enormous and will be manifest throughout your child's life.

2. The first solid foods should be whole foods: cooked squash, carrot, broccoli and other vegetables, avocado, banana, watermelon, etc. Snacks and meals for toddlers and preschoolers should be entirely whole foods. The beverage is water, and that's it, until you find a raw milk source. And even then, the main beverage is water. Toddlers do not need to know that things like pasta and ice cream exist. Parents who exclaim, "But how can I feed them healthy food when macaroni and cheese is the only thing that they'll eat?" have started off with the wrong items in the kitchen, and are going to have to go through some tantrums in order to establish a better way of eating. This will be made easier if you keep your television away from them.

3. TV teaches a processed food and pharmaceutical lifestyle. The messages are delivered continually: either eat out, or open a package to get your ready-made food, pour yourself a glass of colored liquid, and your life is just not happy until you take a pill. If you have to keep de-programming what the TV is programming, you won't be able to compete;

nobody can. TV is so flashy and persuasive that you'll be like Sisyphus always having to roll his rock back up the hill.

Either get rid of the TV, or keep it in a room that always remains locked, to be viewed together only occasionally, when an appropriate movie is to be seen. Kids raised without TV are easily spotted by their teachers. They're the ones with good focus and a longer attention span.

Some families who decide against TV after their kids are already hooked resolve things this way: One day the TV becomes mysteriously "broken," and they just don't get around to buying a new one. Or the TV has to make way for some new bookshelves and ends up on a high shelf in the garage. Anybody who wants to watch it has to go stand next to the car to do so. Suddenly the flashiness loses a lot of its grip on your children's minds.

4. Your children's first friends will tend to be those whose parents you befriend. In other words, almost any two little kids close in age who spend time together will end up playing together, but you are the one who has the discretion to choose your friends wisely. So make your choices of your child's playmates before your child gets around to it. It is very important to your efforts toward a whole food household to bring into your lives moms and dads who are committed to roughly the same kind of diet you are, especially if you also must battle junk-food peddling relatives.

   When your children see others outside of your family eating healthy food, they will understand that it is not just some weird quirk of yours, but that there actually exists a community of like-minded healthy people. When enough of these friends have been gathered into your lives, it will also become obvious to your child that the whole food people look a whole lot healthier than the junk food junkies.

If you don't have a big enough sample size to convince your children of this, take them to the biggest health food store that you know and have them observe the customers. Then take them into a typical supermarket, and have them observe the customers. After you leave, let them discuss comparisons. In which store were people generally heavier and more fatigued-looking? In which store did they see more energetic, moderate weight people of all ages? That kind of powerfully persuasive evidence would even give pause to a teenager who is tempted by fast food eating peers.

5. Keep junk food out of the house. Naturopathic physician Dr. Kenneth Proefrock says the battle over good food is won or lost at the supermarket. If you can walk past processed food at the supermarket and keep on going then you've won. But if cookies made it into your shopping cart, they will make it to your cupboards, and you will end up eating them all and regretting them. Do yourself and your kids a favor. When you're all shopping together, don't even bother going down the processed foods aisles. Shop the periphery where the vegetables, fruits, meats and dairy are, and that's it. Involve your children by letting them make choices among all of those. Pears, peaches or plums? Spinach, mustard greens or romaine? Poultry, fish or red meat? Their choices will be all the tastier when you get home, because each of them got to make those choices.

6. Self-esteem is important to your children's comfort with their diet. Your children also have to participate in social structures involving a majority of children who eat differently. The challenge is to help your children maintain their self-esteem and to honor the food choices of their

> family while also being respectful of others' food choices. All this has to be accomplished with a minimum of awkwardness and isolation. One family shops for mostly organic food, but also at large warehouse supermarkets, where various appetizers are offered to the shoppers around the store. Their five-year old daughter summarized her family's food choices by saying," Look, hot dogs. That's okay, Mommy. We don't eat that. We eat different food, and that's okay too." Regressing from the wisdom of this five-year old, the older child's fear of being different will be fairly calamitous, especially in adolescence, unless there is a strong awareness and self-respect regarding the individual's right to eat differently than most, and the good reasons for doing so.

Talking to your children is the most important. The more that differences become obvious to your children between their diets and others' diets, the more talk is needed. It is very important for your children to know that their healthy lifestyle is at the vanguard of the direction society is moving in, not at the rear. For example, it should be explained to your children that processed food companies are using much less of trans-fatty acids than just a few years ago. Also, fast food chains are offering healthier options now, following their comeuppance from the film "Supersize Me" and other public criticism. School districts are getting continued pressure from parents to disallow soft drink and junk food vending machines in their children's schools. Consistently, a majority of parents surveyed oppose such machines. Now also, a majority of adults surveyed said they would prefer to eat organic food if it were available in their area at a comparable price to non-organic.

Let your children appreciate that your family is way more advanced than many others just because you know how vital it is to eat right. It is gratifying to know that the world is moving in a good direction. Organic food is growing at 12% per year. Even the mighty McDonald's bowed to the public outcry for healthier food. Now your children just need to practice patience as the rest of the world catches up to your trendsetting.

# Chapter 4
# A Birthday Party for a 4-year old . . . without sugar

When my son turned four, he was old enough to have figured out that he must have a birthday party and invite his friends over. So for our first at-home birthday party I invited as many of his little friends and their parents as could squeeze inside our dining room for an evening dinner.

The "cake" is best made as individual mini-cakes, because when you are working with whole foods you are missing some of the textural advantages that grains, particularly refined grains offer. But no worries! It works just fine with little individual cakes made as follows. (This recipe has a lot more appeal for the little ones than the adults generally.)

Cut thick one-inch slices of watermelon.

Then layer in my unsweetened preserves recipe:

3 lbs. fresh or frozen fruit, especially berries of any kind, cut into chunks
3 Granny Smith or other tart apples, peeled and diced (to provide pectin for thickening)
½ tsp pectin powder (optional)

Simmer the berries and apples together over medium heat for about 50 minutes, until boiled down. While fruit is cooking stir often to avoid burning bottom of pan, and mash to aid breakdown of fruit chunks. The apple will need extra mashing to combine thoroughly. Add pectin toward end of cooking. Cool thoroughly before using. (Aside from cake filling, I use this recipe throughout the year to preserve in-season fruit bought in bulk. The preserves can then be canned or frozen, and keep nicely.)

To create layers, start in a small individual bowl with a layer of watermelon. Then layer about a half inch of the cooled preserves. Then top with another layer of watermelon. Finally, layer thin banana slices as the last layer.

If you use watermelon, the finished product will hold candles, which will help hold the layers together. Decorative toothpicks will also help hold everything together. Heavy cream may be poured over the top for an icing-like effect.

A summer-time birthday party for children might include watermelon-only popsicles. These are made by stuffing small chunks of watermelon into popsicle molds and freezing for a couple of hours. Peach and plum chunks also work.

Our birthday party actually began with dinner for the parents and children, a pot roast with vegetables and a salad. The next day, the only thing left over was a chunk of the too-massive pot roast. The cake went over about as well as the pot roast and salad with the restless four and five year olds: the eaters ate quickly; the small-quantity eaters considered eating; the fidgeters fidgeted; and when presents were announced, all food was quickly forgotten about as all of the children rushed into the living room.

Most parents have seen once sweet and obedient children turn into cranky misbehaved rascals after eating sugar. But this party was quite different. It started at 5:00 p.m., and ended around 8:00 p.m., with only one incident of tears after too much roughhousing, and one case of sleepiness. The last hour was actually the most peaceful time, as the children cooperated to quietly complete a big floor puzzle. The parents actually sat and enjoyed relaxed conversation. I think we have all seen social events brought to a halt when kids' behavior becomes intolerable to the point of having to remove them from the party before the evening gets very late. But this good behavior on the part of all the children was enough to make you think, "Gee, if kids can act this good without sugar, then maybe they should never have it at all!"

Those familiar with my online articles may know that my husband and I are raising our son with no sugar or sweeteners at all. But I have to admit that all the children that evening were really angelic, even with very different diets at home. And although most were accustomed to various desserts and sweets, none of the children complained at all about the lack of sweets at our house. This shows me once again that even at the age of 4 or 5 you can remove sugar from your child's diet. Which of course is way easier if your entire household takes the no-sweets plunge together, clearing out every last cookie from the pantry. See the chapters on the sweet tooth.

And the birthday boy? As soon as everybody left at 8:00 p.m., he lay down on the floor and said "Mommy, I want batteries for my new toy. We have to buy batteries today." Then he promptly went to sleep, as he so often ends our nighttime chats.

# Chapter 5
# Junk food in school

Texas Agriculture Commissioner Susan Combs caused a stir at Texas public schools with new rules banning junk food. No sodas or candy bars for gradeschoolers. French fries banned. And bake sale items may not be consumed during school hours. The $104 million that cash-strapped Texas school districts make from junk food sales has corrupted many an administrator. But now, stepping boldly past decades of disgraceful cowardice in the public schools, strewn with the obese, damaged bodies of children, Susan Combs actually has the guts to chase out the junk food dealers. The former prosecutor has little patience with her critics who complain of lost revenue from vending machines and bake sales. "Are we going to sell marijuana to build gyms?" she asks.

Yet there are signs of cooperation. When the Donuts for Dads events were cancelled at Haggar Elementary School in Plano, the parents bought $800 worth of books for the school instead of donuts and other sweets. Snack and soda companies are now falling over themselves trying to devise synthetic "healthy" foods acceptable under the new rules.

As in the rest of the U.S., Texas children have been growing laterally. Over a third are overweight or obese, worse by far than the national rate of 10% to 15% obesity in children. In Texas alone, the estimated cost for treating these kids when they become obese adults is $40 billion. Compounding the problem in Texas, as elsewhere, is the state's inadequate physical education programs and cancelling of recess. "We cram them full of unhealthy food and don't let them expend it. It's a recipe for disaster," says Combs. As for her next project, she plans to address the physical education vacuum.

# Part II
# Surviving a processed food world

# Chapter 6
# The Sweet Tooth, Part I: Defeating the Little Rascal

By now you have probably read enough to understand that sugar and sweets should be crossed off the grocery list. Actually kicking sugar and eliminating cravings is harder, as its many fans know all too well.

As monumental a feat as quitting tobacco is, giving up sugar can be even harder. Most problematic, most people are sugar-addicted, and there is no strong aroma that causes others to chase sugar eaters outdoors, as we do with smokers. This makes eating sweets easy, clean and socially feasible in the home and in public places. Further, the social isolation of smokers has forced them to acknowledge their addiction and the difficulties that tobacco creates in a smoker's life. But the showering of sugar on our children, and as a result our almost universal addiction to sugar allows a comfortable blanket of denial to settle over our minds and lifestyles, blinding us to the growing problems accumulating in our arteries, heart, nervous system, kidneys and other internal organs. Sugar is not seen as a public health problem, although it is the most relentless, widespread and entrenched one.

What makes giving up sugar even harder though is the many different methods proposed by the various experts. Most famously, Dr. Robert Atkins advised to simply give up sugar and other high-carbohydrate foods altogether, while consoling oneself for the loss with unlimited high-fat and high-protein foods. This diet has worked miraculously for many people. Yet for many others, large quantities of proteins and fats are not digestible or appropriate for their metabolic type.[19] Dr. Barry Sears' *The Zone* offers some simple sugars in the diet along with mostly healthier foods, but this simply keeps the addiction going, and does not heal the main problem of sugar cravings. Dr. Arthur Agatston's *The South Beach Diet* urges minimizing sweets, but also includes such items as ice cream and bread, which contribute to the long-term torture of a frequently teased addiction. A similar problem occurs with *The Carbohydrate Addict's Diet* by Drs. Rachael and Richard Heller, in which a "reward meal" is available in the evening to those who have denied their sugar cravings during the day. This also keeps a sugar addiction regularly fueled and stoked, ultimately resulting in frustration for the trusting dieter. These diets are as defeating in the long run for the sugar consumer as one cigarette a day – for years – is for the smoker.

Writers such as William Dufty, *Sugar Blues* and Nancy Appleton, *Lick the Sugar Habit*, have dealt with the problem of sugar addiction by advising the reader of the medical horrors of long-term sugar

---

[19] Metabolic typing is described and illustrated in its impact on an individual's wellbeing by William Wolcott and Dr. Joseph Mercola on the website and newsletter Mercola.com, which is the largest of the alternative health websites. http://www.mercola.com/2002/dec/18/metabolic_typing.htm.

consumption, and by advocating complete avoidance. The diets exclude sugars, and Dr. Appleton advocates chromium and glutamine supplements to replenish the sugar-ravaged body and to stabilize sugar cravings. Another workable diet, which is less well-known than most of the preceding works, is *The Sugar Addict's Total Recovery Program*, by Kathleen DesMaisons, Ph.D., in which the dieter works in stages, going "slow carb" first before "low carb". Slow carbs are those that are accompanied by a lot of fiber or protein, which slow down the entry of sugar to the bloodstream. That is, at first substituting whole grain bread for white bread, steel-cut oats for other cereals, sweets with protein for sweets alone, and similar substitutions makes the important first step of taking the sugar addict from the glucose-insulin roller coaster of extreme highs and lows to a more moderate fluctuation of biochemicals and hence moods and feelings. Once in the more moderate rhythm of blood analytes, the dieter is in a much stronger position to handle a reduction, then elimination of simple sugars. In Des Maisons' book, the last cold-turkey withdrawal is still a bit of a cliff jump, but she certainly strengthens the dieter toward that end.

The final step of giving up sugar with the help of chromium supplementation has been established as beneficial.[20] It is also useful for the dieter to understand which other nutrients are affected by high sugar states and low sugar states (both of which are visited by the sugar addict on a daily basis), and to know how to substitute healthier foods that contain those same needed nutrients.

For example, sugar cravings and sugar rebound involve deficiencies of the following nutrients:

[20] Chromium picolinate supplementation at 1,000mcg per day for a 13-week period together with exercise lowered total cholesterol, LDL cholesterol and insulin levels in a study of both males and females. J Nutr Biochem, 1998;9: pp.471-5.

Chromium, which may be found in broccoli, cheese, dried beans, calf liver and chicken;

Carbon, which may be found in fresh fruits;

Phosphorus, which may be found in chicken, beef, liver, poultry, fish, eggs, dairy, nuts and legumes;

Sulphur, which may be found in onions, garlic, cranberries, horseradish and cruciferous vegetables;

And tryptophan, which may be found in cheese, liver, lamb and spinach.

In the case of chocolate cravings, magnesium is also deficient, and may be found in raw nuts and seeds, legumes and fruits.[21] [22]

Dr. Decker Weiss, a medical school lecturer and naturopathic cardiologist, memorably informed us in Cardiology class one day, "If you want heart disease, eat a pastry; it's got everything you need: sugar, flour and trans-fatty acids." His book, *The Weiss Method*, is a program in stages for overcoming unhealthy cravings with healthy food substitutions, while bringing his expertise in both cardiology and the vastly eclectic naturopathic medicine to focus on improving the health of his patients.

Ultimately, the way to win the eating game is to choose the healthiest foods possible in the widest variety available, with respect to your metabolic type. However, for the sugarholic, some extra care with the above substitutions will be a necessary component of breaking the chains of sugar addiction.

---

[21] Lectures, Cheryl M. Deroin, N.M.D., Southwest College of Naturopathic Medicine, Tempe, AZ. Spring, 2003 (healthy food recommendations).

[22] Bernard Jensen, Ph.D., The Chemistry of Man, B. Jensen Publisher, 1983. (deficiencies linked to specific cravings and some food recommendations)

# Chapter 7
# The Sweet Tooth, Part 2: More Deprivation Caused By Regular Pampering

If you've got a sweet tooth, you know that it doesn't let you ignore it for very long. At least once every day or two, the boss lets you know who's in charge. You rummage around the kitchen for sweets, check all the way to the back of the refrigerator; dart out to the store if necessary. A sense of sugar/chocolate deprivation sets in, and demands that you do something about it. Not that the sweet tooth can be calmed down for weeks at a time by an especially large dessert or other massive binge. Wouldn't that be convenient!

Why does this happen? How does a person who regularly indulges the sweet tooth end up feeling more deprived - and more frequently deprived - than those insufferable serene types who don't eat sweets? It has to do with a process called homeostasis. When you eat a lot of sugar, your body notes that your blood glucose level is higher than normal. As a result, the pancreas secretes insulin, which packs this sugar away into cells that process it, in order to bring your blood sugar back to normal. When a lot of sugar is ingested, a lot of insulin comes out and packs it all away, which overcompensates and swings your blood sugar too low for a while. This accounts for the afternoon brain fog (transient hypoglycemia) often experienced after a high-carbohydrate lunch. And this is when the sweet tooth (really, just a euphemism for a sugar habit plus a fluctuating blood glucose) wakes up and reminds you who's really boss.

It doesn't have to be this way, of course. Sugar cravings like all other cravings can be overcome by substituting better quality, but equally satisfactory, foods. You just have to know exactly what kinds of good foods can satisfy which kinds of urges. Cravings are actually the manifestation of a mild malnutrition, which is very widespread, even in well-to-do societies. We will go into this at length in Chapter 11.

So we end up craving the vitamins and especially minerals that we lack. But while your body may know that you are missing for example magnesium, your conscious mind is not aware of the flavor of magnesium. Instead, because of familiarity, you can reminisce and feel hungry for the flavor of chocolate, which is high in magnesium, and which has its appeal partly rooted in its magnesium. The chocolate that your conscious mind desires has its greatest ability to quench those cravings due to chocolate's high magnesium content.

Of course, the sugar in commercially prepared chocolate is another desperate desire when you have ridden the sugar-insulin roller coaster long enough to plummet to the abyss of hypoglycemia. The food cravings of PMS are due to poor glucose tolerance brought on by diets that are high in refined carbohydrates. Refined sugars deplete the body's supplies of B-vitamins, chromium, magnesium, zinc and manganese, and the resulting deficiencies then manifest as cravings for other foods. What adds insult to injury here is that whole sugar cane is actually high in these minerals. In fact, of all known plants, the one with the highest known proportion of chromium is, of all things, sugar cane. Chromium is necessary for insulin function and to modulate blood sugar levels. Then the refining process strips out the minerals, so that the whole food, which nature put together so wisely, now becomes something that destroys our health, heaves our blood sugar and blood insulin into wildly gyrating chaos, and leaves us craving what the refining process threw away.

This simply adds to the mountain of evidence that nature knew what she was doing when she made whole food. This is not to say that sugar cane or the minimally processed molasses should be consumed. The torture of the huge sugar-insulin assault on your pancreas and liver and brain is really not worth the minerals gained from eating it. Those minerals are available from healthier sources.

**Fruit: not just another sweetener**

People often ask, "Isn't fruit just as bad for you as desserts with refined carbohydrates and concentrated sweeteners?" Definitely not! Refined carbohydrates, such as sugar and flour are only fragments from original whole foods that contained all of the molecules necessary for their optimal digestion. What's left by the time it's packaged and sold to you as a dessert is something quite different, an artery-slathering, fiberless, nutrient-robbed shadow of its former self.

Fruit on the other hand has the fiber necessary to slow down the entry of natural sugars to the bloodstream, which keeps your insulin at moderate levels. Insulin is what is particularly important not to let spike too high. Some fruits are better at this than others. For example, bananas and papayas tend to spike blood sugar and insulin, more than apples, because in apples the natural sugars are slowed down by the accompanying fiber. Another advantage of fruit is that it has not been stripped of its inherent vitamins, minerals and enzymes, many of which are necessary for its complete digestion.

# Chapter 8
# The Sweet Tooth, Part 3: Sugar cravings and candida

Yeasts, such as candida, feed on sugar. Women with recurrent vaginal yeast infections may begin to feel as if candida is a permanent fixture of their bodies, and indeed we can carry it with us all our lives. That does not mean, however, that candida has to be in control of your life. John Parks Trowbridge, MD and Morton Walker, authors of The Yeast Syndrome, are medical mavericks in their diagnosis and treatment of yeast complications that their conventional medical colleagues insisted could not exist, because they had never been taught about them. Yet time has shown that Trowbridge, Walker, and other health professionals who have worked with candida patients have accurately identified a relentless and ubiquitous pathogen in the common *Candida albicans,* along with the many havoc-wreaking antibodies that it generates.

Trowbridge and Walker have found patients mostly improving completely in about ten days. But very tenacious cases may need up to three years before completely recovery of symptoms. Naturopathic physician Dr. Leslie Axelrod in Scottsdale, AZ uses an eating plan that deprives candida of its fuel of choice: sugar. Melons, mushrooms and other foods are also limited for a time. The duration of this diet corresponds to the severity of the symptoms, varies somewhat according to individual needs, and is generally followed for as long as the patient continues to have symptoms.

The hard part of this diet for someone with a heavy candida load is eliminating sugar, since the candida in the body is screaming for sugar. Since eliminating sugar is a huge step in your life, it merits advance planning and preparation. Start modulating your blood sugar by switching some sweets to complex carbohydrates including whole vegetables. Supplements such as glutamine (an amino acid sold in sports nutrition-type stores), fenugreek, chromium and other nutrients are used by naturopathic physicians to help their patients eliminate sugar cravings. It is best to use these while in the care of a naturopathic physician, in order to choose the most appropriate of the available forms and for correct dosing and combinations.

Not all of these need be used. It is important when quitting sugar to remember that your body is fighting as hard to overcome these cravings as a heroin addict feels during withdrawal or a smoker trying to quit. (Actually, nicotine is the most addictive of the three, and aren't you glad you don't have to quit *that* !) This also means that the worst part will be the first 48 hours of abstinence. After that, it definitely gets better. The first two weeks will be a little less comfortable than afterward, but the reward for persisting is that after two weeks you will feel healthier in every way than you have ever felt.

Those who quit extremely addictive substances say that it is more effective to affirm "I will not eat sugar today," rather than say, "I will never eat sugar again," which is too daunting. Just affirm each day that you will not have sugar that day, which breaks up your job into manageable pieces.

Also, henceforth, you are not allowed to own, borrow, taste or have in your possession any sugar or sweets. Feel free to inform any sugar-offering person that this is your contractual agreement with me, the author of this book.

To get through moment-to-moment cravings, you can massage all of both ears, in order to cover the acupuncture points for addiction. Also, take a few slow deep breaths. Greater success is likely if you convince your entire household to take a sugar-free plunge with you. That way you can keep temptation out of your house, which is 90% of the battle. Finally, get involved in a new hobby or activity, preferably one that involves the hands, such as art, music, gardening, etc. in order to help get through the first two days successfully.

### Candida's stealth invasion of the human body

Fungi such as candida can cause problems as diverse as frequent bouts of colds or athlete's foot or urinary tract infections or PMS or irritable bowel or "brain fog". Chronic sinusitis is another condition that researchers are finding may have to do with chronic fungal infection in the nose. See a recent Mayo Clinic sinusitis study at http://www.stopyeast.com/sinusitis.html

One does not need to suffer from all of these conditions to have a candida problem; different people have different susceptibilities, which means that you and I could both have candida, but I get a chronic athlete's foot infection, and you get a rumbly abdomen instead, manifesting completely different reactions to this same organism. Most invading pathogens have more recognizable patterns of disrupting the human body. Some go to the urinary system, some to the lungs, some to the GI tract, etc. Candida is a complicated and systemic pathogen. It weakens our immune system, which often allows other body systems to be attacked by other opportunistic microbes such as bacteria and viruses.

# Chapter 9
# Artificial Sweeteners

Both the FDA and the American Medical Association have pronounced aspartame to be safe. Sweetening sodas, candies, gum and other processed foods for a quarter century, it has been consumed by many people who show no obvious symptoms. Then, on the other hand, there are the people who have consumed enough aspartame over time that they have ended up with symptoms of multiple sclerosis. A number of other diseases, otherwise unexplained, have followed aspartame use. These include: grand mal seizures,[23] migraines and exacerbation of pre-

[23] Wurtman R. Aspartame: possible effect on seizure susceptibility. Lancet 1985 Nov 9. No. 2 (8463):1060.

existing migraines,[24] urticaria, and granulomatosis[25] A powerful neurotoxin, aspartame has been listed by the Pentagon as an agent of chemical warfare.[26]

Dr. Alan Gaby warns that subtle reactions to aspartame may also be common, and that it should be suspect in patients with various vague or unexplained symptoms.

Our taste buds have been conditioned to the far extreme of the sweet end of the spectrum of tastes. This has cost us heavily in terms of either sugar use and its many undesirable consequences, or the perhaps even worse damage caused by artificial sweeteners. Dr. Gaby challenges his patients to avoid both and allow their taste buds "to be reawakened to the natural sweet taste of whole foods." [27]

Adverse effects of aspartame also include: brain tumors, epilepsy, Parkinson's disease, chronic fatigue syndrome, fibromyalgia and Alzheimer's, among many other neurological disorders and illnesses. 90 different documented symptoms have been reported in humans. The way that aspartame works is that it allows a very large influx of calcium into neurons, which produce overexcitement to the point of killing the neuron. For this reason, aspartame and similar chemicals are called excitotoxins.

Sucralose, another popular artificial sweetener has been successfully marketed as natural sweetener, with the claim that it is derived from sugar. This part is true; however, the molecule is

---

[24] Koehler, S et al. The effect of aspartame on migraine headache. Headache 1988. No. 28.
[25] Reed B et al. Orofacial sensitivity reactions and the role of dietary components. Case reports. Ast Dent J. 1993. No. 38.
[26] http://www.mercola.com/article/aspartame/fraud.htm
[27] Gaby, A. Is Aspartame safe? (editorial). Townsend Letter. May, 2005

so radically changed to form the artificial sweetener that it has little resemblance to sugar.

You may have loved ones with a diet soda habit. As you approach them about making healthier substitutions, they will put up a little defensive wall, which has written on it "everything in moderation." Then they will argue that only one (or two) diet sodas everyday is a moderate amount. However, toxic effects of aspartame have been produced at amounts much less than in one can of soda.

But regular soda is not a good choice either. Soda contains phosphoric acid, which has a pH of 2.8. Phosphoric acid also leaches calcium out of bones, and is a major factor in the rising incidence of osteoporosis. Give your body a break: drink water instead.

# Chapter 10
# The Bread Trap

Bread is a vehicle. In a sandwich, it drives other food neatly and with little spillage into a bag or wrapper, into a lunchbox and then to the mouth. Popular at drive-ins, the sandwich can be sort of neatly eaten with one hand while the other hand sort of competently manages the steering wheel. Bread envelops; it absorbs excess liquids; it shapes the contents within for optimal handling. And that's just for lunch.

Later, at dinner, when eating tends to be somewhat more formal, with possibly some sauce or other potential messiness, sitting on a plate, there is sometimes a desire to wipe up the last drop of liquid with an edible sponge. Again bread serves a purpose.

Lightweight, dry, fresh enough at room temperature at least for a while, bread transports well, and sits neatly on a shelf. No wonder that bread, or similar wheat products, sweetened or plain, is ubiquitous throughout much of the world and the darling of the processed food industry, in one of its many forms: loaf, bagel, donut, muffin, pasta, croissant, frybread, roll, birthday cake. In these sweetened forms, bread and other wheat flour products are among the most common breakfast foods.

So for the many years that USDA's food pyramid was dead-weighted with the absurdly large 11 servings of grains and grain products, both the government and the average person took the satire of a diet seriously, and actually ate up all that bread and brought it into every meal, not to mention snacks.

Wheat cultivation had spread from the Fertile Crescent of the Middle East through much of the world by 4,000 BC, which until modern food distribution and storage was developed, played an essential role in sustaining populations through long periods between harvests when there was no other food. This in turn enabled nomadic hunter-gatherers to settle into permanent communities and to even trade away excess wheat with outsiders. Wheat's utility in the problem of seasonal famines has ensured its continual increase in acreage until the present day, when it has reached a peak of cultivated acreage. Increasing yields per acre and population rates that are not rising as fast as before have now led to a stabilized acreage under cultivation for wheat.

However, the wheat that our ancestors ate was different in form, quantity and antigenicity from what people eat today. Until the 19th century, a very recent time in human history, wheat was generally mixed with other grains, beans and nuts. Only in the last 200 years has a pure wheat flour with a high gluten content been milled to the point of refined white flour. Generally, the wheat that people eat is no longer stone ground from whole meal flour, as even our recent ancestors ate. By now, almost all of us alive today have been given white wheat flour products on a daily basis from a few months of age – before the intestinal lining can properly filter anything other than mother's milk to the bloodstream.

**So now it's too late**

Even if an individual attempts to eliminate all grain from the diet except for stone ground grain, it's too late. The high-gluten, refined grain that we have all eaten from infancy has created a ubiquitous problem from the gut to the bloodstream to the brain and sometimes to the joints, cardiovascular system and endocrine system as well. The food sensitivity that our food culture has dropped on us has done the kind of damage that leaves no easily identifying marks. Bread inflicts wounds so subtly and gradually that most of us consider ourselves immune to any such damage.

The huge and complex gluten protein, and especially its gliadin fraction, is thought to be the worst problem in the gluten-containing grains. The proportion of gluten in wheat has been enormously increased by hybridization since our distant ancestors first started making food from the wild grasses. Gluten is from the Greek word for glue, and its adhesive, elastic property is the very thing that holds the bread loaf or bite of cake together. But when that glue hits the intestines, it interferes with the breakdown and absorption of nutrients in the accompanying foods of the same meal. And because it is of almost no nutritional value itself – nutrients having been bred out in favor of the more marketable adhesive properties - little value is gained from that meal. At best, even the person who considers himself immune to wheat allergy, is getting a worthless glued-together constipating lump in the gut from what was considered a nourishing meal. At best, a run-down, mildly fatigued feeling is a constant symptom of the adult with the fewest reactions to wheat. And we actually ruin every meal of the day with one of the most antigenic foods on the planet.

At worst, such diseases as rheumatoid arthritis, lupus, multiple sclerosis and cancers such as lymphoma can result from severe celiac disease or extreme gluten sensitivity. In between are many who may have occasional unexplained diarrhea or intestinal gas and bloating, vague joint pains, infertility or brain fog.

In order to effectively replace wheat you're going to have to find a way to accomplish some of what the adhesive/elastic properties of wheat flour do. A sandwich thus becomes a lettuce wrap. Or its contents are placed on a plate or in a bowl. Meats, vegetables and fruits play a more prominent role. A spoon is ready to scoop up the last of the sauce on the dinner plate.

You can make a lot of extra work for yourself by going to the supermarket and attempting to replace all of the breads and desserts in a typical diet with gluten-free grains, but you're still getting a nutritionally depleted meal – poor compensation for spending extra time reading processed food packages for which have gluten and which do not. The whole food solution is the simplest and most nourishing. Shop the produce aisle and the meat aisle, and let those purchases alone comprise your diet. It will make you discover new and delicious vegetables that you have never tried before, and it will get you out of the bread trap.

# Chapter 11
# "Everything in moderation" is a recipe for disaster

A favorite mantra is "everything in moderation." On the surface it sounds quite reasonable, avoiding fanatical or extreme activities by the very definition of moderation. Reasonable people are moderate. Good parents and teachers are moderate, aren't they? So what could be the problem with it?

Actually, consuming everything in moderation is not very healthy at all. This is primarily because most foods available today are of such poor quality that their net effect is as much harm as good, as much toxicity as nutrition. Supermarkets are mostly stocked with foods laced with chemicals that are biologically disruptive as well as refined carbohydrates and the many products that contain them. The whole natural foods are relatively marginalized in supermarkets, off in the produce aisle and all the way in the back with the meats. Even then there are few or no organic foods, and the meats are full of hormones, pesticides, antibiotics and other substances that disrupt the immune system, the neurological system, the endocrine system, and that generally do not belong in the human body.

The result is that a moderate sampling of everything in the store leaves a shopper with:

- almost all pesticide-laden foods
- most foods containing refined carbohydrates
- most foods containing MSG (monosodium glutamate) or one of its many aliases, such as hydrolyzed whey protein, or other equally unhealthy neurotoxic additives, such as disodium inosinate, maltodextrin, autolyzed yeast extract, etc.

Pesticides are not something you want in your body. Organic farmers eating organic food were found to have normal sperm, while their conventional counterparts eating non-organic food did not. Many pesticides were correlated with dead or defective sperm.[28] Pesticide consumption is also linked with stillbirth[29] as well as development of Parkinson's Disease,[30] aggressive behavior and irritability[31]. Of the 25 most commonly used agricultural pesticides:

18 can damage the skin, eyes and lungs,

---

[28] Juhler R, et al. Human semen quality in relation to dietary pesticide exposure and organic diet. Arch Environ Contam Toxicol 1999; 37:415-423.
[29] Occupational and Environmental Medicine. 1997. 54; 511-518.
[30] Annual Meeting of the American Academy of Neurology in San Diego. May 9, 2000.
[31] Rachel's Environment and Health Weekly, #648, April 29,1999. (See article in Mercola.com.)

17 cause genetic damage or birth defects,
12 cause cancer,
10 cause reproductive problems,
6 disrupt normal hormone function.

5 are neurotoxins,[32] which is the most common harm shown clinically in those whose only contact with pesticides is food consumption.

But it is not only fruits and vegetables that are contaminated with pesticides. In fact, meat and dairy concentrate pesticides much more, especially in the fat tissue of farm animals. The EPA concluded in 1992 that Americans were exposed to 300 to 600 times the "acceptable" level of the toxic chemical dioxin every day in food and water. Chicken, eggs, red meat, fish and dairy products were the most frequently contaminated foods.[33] Another pesticide, Dursban, was found in the urine of over 90% of Minnesota school children. Dursban has been a known cause of birth defects and cancer for many years. Yet it is still found in at least 22 foods tested by the USDA.[34]

And everything discussed here so far is within the scope of a "moderate" diet; no extreme binging or food faddism. But there's more:

Every day nine of 10 children aged six months to five years are exposed to combinations of 13 different nerve-damaging

[32] Rapp, Doris. Our Toxic World: A Wake Up Call. Environmental Medical Research Foundation. 2004.
[33] Ibid.
[34] ibid.

insecticides in the food they eat, even after washing and processing the food.[35] [36]

It is really imperative for your health that you begin to eat organic produce right away. But it is even more urgent that your meat and dairy be organic. If supermarkets near you don't have it, demand it. If they still won't get it, become a local weekend distributor yourself.

Some organic wholesalers are: The New Farm, Organic Valley, or check out BlueSky Search for a large list of organic food wholesalers. These can all be found on the internet. A few signs put up in your neighborhood will bring out all kinds of like-minded people you never new existed. Start small, out of your garage or front porch on Saturday mornings. Start with a few in-season fruits and vegetables. Later when you get a lot of regular subscribing members, and some favorable articles written about you in your local newspaper, you can rent out warehouse space and expand and maybe even make that your day job.

As for refined carbohydrates, even small amounts of these reinforce addiction to them, refresh your candida while fatiguing you, stress your adrenals, pancreas and brain, and give you nothing in return. They are the emptiest of empty calories, as Dr. Atkins called them. He had a rule for determining how much refined carbs you could have in moderation. "Take a piece of paper. Take a pencil. Draw a large circle on the paper. Read the answer. That's a zero."[37] So much for moderation.

---

[35] Wiles R. et al. Overexposed: organophosphate insecticides in children's food. Environmental Working Group. Washington. January, 1998.

[36] An excellent, thoroughly researched work on this topic is Doris Rapp MD's book Our Toxic World: A Wake Up Call.

[37] Atkins, Robert, MD. Dr. Atkins' Age-Defying Diet. St. Martins Press. New York. 2001.

# Chapter 12
# If you crave this . . .

Food cravings can seem strong enough to pick you up and carry you straight to the refrigerator or convenience store independent of your will and better judgment. For many women, cravings are especially intense in the week or so before menstruation. But many men, older women, teens and children can have strong cravings too. Let's look at what is behind this force. Naturopathic physician Tori Hudson, ND, describes the condition as a mild malnutrition, certainly not with severe overt consequences as say scurvy or rickets. Rather, a great many people on the Standard American Diet (SAD in more ways than one) suffer from a milder malnutrition from eating only depleted, processed foods and not enough whole, nutrient-rich foods.

As a result, we end up craving the vitamins, minerals and other nutrients that we lack. But while your body may know that you are missing for example potassium, your conscious mind is not aware of the flavor of potassium. Instead, because of familiarity, you can reminisce and feel hungry for the flavor of salty foods, which are high in another cation, sodium, and which have their appeal partly rooted in sodium and potassium. The salty foods that your conscious mind desires has its greatest ability to quench those cravings due to the salty foods' high sodium content.

So how do you wrap yourself around healthier food choices if you have never eaten healthy food? Steven Ehrlich, ND, an Arizona naturopathic physician recommends starting very slowly and gradually. He likes to add, rather than subtract, from his patient's diets. For example, he might instruct the patient to add an apple every day. Once that's going well and has become a habit, they might later add some salmon, then a salad. As the healthy items start filling up the menu and the patient's tummy, the highly processed foods begin falling away surreptitiously as they get replaced. Gradually, the patient is encouraged to continue to improve the diet by the rewarding health benefits that accrue to those who eat well. This is probably the most painless way to clean up the diet, provided the patient is steadfast and sticks with it permanently.

The bottom line is: the way to win the eating game is to choose the healthiest foods possible in the widest variety available, with respect to your metabolic type.[38] The following table gives the best food options for overcoming various kinds of cravings.

---

[38] See the Chapter on metabolic type.

*If you crave this . . .* © *Colleen Huber, NMD*
http://www.naturopathyworks.com/

| ***If you crave this . . .*** | ***Then what you really want and need is this . . .*** | ***And here are healthy foods that have it: (listed in order of benefit).. Please note that <u>everyone</u> needs a wide variety of whole fresh foods and to minimize refined, sweetened and processed "foods" in the diet*** |
|---|---|---|
| **Chocolate** | **Magnesium** | **Raw nuts and seeds, legumes, fruits** |
| **Sweets** | **Chromium** | **Broccoli, grapes, cheese, dried beans, calf liver, chicken** |
| | **Carbon** | **Fresh fruits** |
| | **Phosphorus** | **Chicken, beef, liver, poultry, fish, eggs, dairy, nuts, legumes** |
| | **Sulphur** | **Cranberries, horseradish, cruciferous vegetables: kale, cabbage** |

| | | |
|---|---|---|
| | Tryptophan | Cheese, liver, lamb, raisins, sweet potatoes, spinach |
| Bread, toast | Nitrogen | High protein foods: fish, meat, nuts, beans |
| Oily snacks, fatty foods | Calcium | Mustard and turnip greens, broccoli, kale, legumes, cheese, sesame |
| Coffee or tea | Phosphorus | Chicken, beef, liver, poultry, fish, eggs, dairy, nuts, legumes |
| | Sulphur | Egg yolks, red peppers, muscle protein, garlic, onion, cruciferous vegetables |
| | HCl | Sea salt, apple cider vinegar on your salads |
| | Iron | Meat, fish and poultry, seaweed, greens, black cherries |
| Alcohol, recreational drugs | Protein | Meat, poultry, seafood, dairy, nuts |
| | Avenin (a protein found in oats) | Oatmeal, granola |

| | | |
|---|---|---|
| | **Calcium** | **Mustard and turnip greens, broccoli, kale, legumes, cheese, sesame** |
| | **Glutamine** | **Supplement glutamine powder for acute withdrawal; raw cabbage juice** |
| | **Potassium** | **Sun-dried black olives, potato peel broth, seaweed, bitter greens** |
| **Chewing on ice** | **Iron** | **Meat, fish and poultry, seaweed, greens, black cherries** |

| Burned food | Carbon | Fresh fruits |
|---|---|---|
| Soda/ Carbonated drinks | Calcium | Mustard and turnip greens, broccoli, kale, legumes, cheese, sesame |
| Salty foods | Chloride | Raw goat milk, fish. Use sea salt, not refined. |
| Acid foods | Magnesium | Raw nuts and seeds, legumes, fruits |
| Liquids more than solids | Water | Flavor water with lemon or lime to make it tastier. You *need* 8 – 10 glasses per day. |
| Solids but not liquids | Water | You have been so dehydrated for so long, that you have lost your thirst. Flavor water with lemon or lime to make it more palatable. |
| Cool drinks | Manganese | Walnuts, almonds, pecans, pineapple, blueberries |
| Pre-menstrual cravings | Zinc | Red meats, esp. organ meats, seafood, vegetables: leafy and root |

| | | |
|---|---|---|
| Overeating in general | Silicon | Nuts, seeds; avoid refined starches |
| | Tryptophan | Cheese, liver, lamb, raisins, sweet potatoes, spinach |
| | Tyrosine | Vitamin C supplement or from orange, green and red fruits and vegetables |
| Lack of appetite | Vitamin B-1 | Nuts, seeds, beans, liver and other organ meats |
| | Vitamin B-3 | Tuna, halibut, beef, chicken, turkey, pork, seeds and legumes |
| | Manganese | Walnuts, almonds, pecans, pineapple, blueberries |
| | Chloride | Raw goat milk, fish. Use sea salt, not refined. |
| Tobacco | Silicon | Nuts, seeds; avoid refined starches |

| | | |
|---|---|---|
| | **Tyrosine** | **Vitamin C supplement or from orange, green and red fruits and vegetables** |

Sources:

1. Lectures, Cheryl M. Deroin, N.M.D., Southwest College of Naturopathic Medicine, Tempe, AZ. Spring, 2003 (healthy food recommendations)
2. Bernard Jensen, Ph.D., The Chemistry of Man, B. Jensen Publisher, 1983. (deficiencies linked to specific cravings and some food recommendations)

# Chapter 13
# Blood type, Metabolic type and your own type

Dr. Peter D'Adamo, a naturopathic physician working from his own research and that of his father, developed a widely respected system of determining optimal diet by looking at one's blood type. Dr. D'Adamo observed that distant ancestral origins and migratory patterns are seen in historical patterns of blood type. People of a given blood type tend to have a common ancestry regarding food: hunter-gatherer or agrarian, etc. Type O, being the oldest, is that descended mostly from hunter-gatherers, while the newer blood types, A, B and AB tend to have more agricultural and pastoral backgrounds. As a result, the various blood types, the D'Adamos observed, vary from each other in the optimal diet for each of them

Metabolic typing was developed by Dr. William Wolcott[39]. He also observed that one's ancestral origins determined the optimal diet for the descendants. For example, the Inuit have an almost completely carnivorous diet, yet heart disease and cancer are unheard of among them. Their language lacks words for those diseases. At the opposite end of the food spectrum, the East Indians have a completely vegetarian diet and enjoy great health. The Swiss have traditional diets very high in dairy, without the dairy problems that other nationalities have had with dairy. Therefore, an Inuit who attempts vegetarianism may fare poorly as would an East Indian attempting the carnivorous Inuit diet.

Individual typing is also an option, and especially useful because individuals don't all fit into the exact stereotype for their blood type or nationality. For example, an individual who was fed wheat too early in life (before 6-8 months) often shows sensitivity to wheat. Such a reaction could manifest in many different ways. In celiac disease (extreme wheat intolerance), the child is severely underweight and may even fail to thrive. There are lesser degrees of wheat intolerance, which is usually an intolerance toward the gluten part of the wheat. These may manifest as leaky gut syndrome, a tendency to malabsorption of nutrients or gas and bloating. The skin and central nervous system are also commonly affected.

Such individual diet analysis can be accomplished with a blood draw. Your naturopathic physician can send this in for laboratory analysis. Your blood can then be checked for over 100 foods, with a list prepared for you of those foods that you reacted to, and those that are more tolerable for you. Such individualized typing can short cut months to years of experimenting with different foods.

---

[39] Wolcott, William. The Metabolic Typing Diet

In addition, food sensitivities can take from 4 to 14 days to clear from the body, making it almost impossible to pinpoint a specific food that you may have eaten days ago as being causative of your symptoms.

Any of these diets is a good way to start and will give you the means to start feeling better and reducing symptoms.

# Chapter 14
# How To Cook Whole Food From Scratch—and Keep Your Day Job!

Whole fresh foods should be the basis of what we all eat, whether one's metabolic type is Protein Type, Carb Type or Mixed Type. Whole foods, whether meat, vegetable or fruit, do two things: they provide all the nutrients that nature put into the food – not just as a sum of nutrients, but even more, as a synergy of nutrients that work together because they naturally interact within the living plant or animal. When we eat these foods, which have been connected with our whole existence as a species, the total health benefit to us of these nutrients working together is much greater than the sum of the parts. The second practical advantage of eating whole fresh foods is that they substitute, by their sheer bulk, the chemicals and denatured food derivatives that we might otherwise eat.

But you work non-stop and when you get home there is no time or energy to do anything but nuke half-synthetic processed food in the microwave. How do we get into that trap?

According to Dr. Kenneth Proefrock, NMD, a huge part of the problem is not knowing what you're going to eat on Thursday night until . . . Thursday night. By that time, you're lucky if you even make it home for dinner because your tummy rang the dinner bell back around Exit 128, and there just happen to be about four fast food outlets off that exit, as well as at the next exit coming up. (Funny how those fast food places are right there when the stomach growls.)

Here's a big key, says Dr. Proefrock, to getting out of that trap. Plan on the weekend what you will eat for every meal the coming week. Your menu does not have to be set in stone; you can leave room to juggle for spontaneity now and then, but at least provide for enough of your own homemade food to eat each time you get hungry.

So how do you make your own homemade whole food and keep your day job too?

Here are several steps you can take to streamline your efforts, and maximize the productivity of your kitchen, while keeping to a minimum your time spent there.

1) Clear enough freezer space, about one cubic foot, to store several pint and quart-size containers of the food you will cook. Then on the weekend, plan all of your meals for the week, and go to the supermarket once to purchase the

whole food ingredients in one trip. Consolidating all grocery shopping into one trip already saves time over shopping for a few items everyday. Plus, with whole foods, you only need to go around the periphery of the supermarket where they are located, rather than taking time to go up and down all of the interior aisles where the processed foods are.

2) Once you've brought home all the groceries, cook all your meals for the week at the same time. This way, instead of standing at the stovetop each day for each meal, you are there for one longer session during that week, and then you're done! The trick is to *cook big portions, but refrigerate and freeze in the smaller quantities that you and your family will eat throughout the week.* If you cook for a family, a large recipe will probably be good for two dinners (on alternate days) during the week, as well as a lunch or two. If you live alone, you will get at least four meal portions, with half of them saved for the following week. At this point you don't have to spend any more time throughout the week than you would on TV dinners.

3) A food processor will work well for foods that you want to chop finely. Make freezer bags full of pre-cut vegetables that you can then defrost as needed during the week. One bag might contain finely minced garlic with coarsely chopped string beans, which a few days from now you can sauté in olive oil for a few minutes. Another bag might contain chopped carrots, onions and tomatoes, along with cabbage that you cut into quarters. Sprinkle some caraway seeds into the bag. When you're ready to make a meal of it, you can cook it in a cup of chicken broth for a delicious meal of balanced nutrients.

4) Make use of large cooking vessels in order to accomplish the weekend cooking fiesta. A large crockpot really lends itself well to a whole foods diet. Here you don't need a food processor. Chop vegetables very coarsely, in much larger chunks than you can get away with in a stovetop meal. This step alone saves the most time if chopping by hand. Put a beef round or two turkey legs or a whole chicken on top of the vegetables, add a few cups of water, and/or tomato sauce, perhaps with balsamic vinegar. Sesame oil and/or tamari may be used instead for marinade. Add whole leaf herbs as you like, and you're done. After practicing once or twice, you will have a huge crockpot meal thrown together in 5-10 minutes. Set it on "low" in the morning, and you're done till dinnertime. In cool weather, you could do the same in the regular oven, with a Dutch oven type covered pot in one and a half hours.

5) Now it's a Tuesday morning, and you'll need something for dinner. Defrost one of the meals you prepared on the weekend. In the evening when you're ready to cook it, place it into a serving dish in a toaster oven rather than a microwave. Toaster ovens have several advantages over microwaves. At about $40 they are much cheaper, smaller, and quieter. However, those benefits are far outweighed by the health advantage: microwave rays are unhealthy radiation, and when you microwave in a plastic container, it drives the phthalates of the plastic right into your food, which gives an otherwise excellent meal a toxic twist that you definitely do not need. Microwave radiation also leaks throughout the whole kitchen from most microwave ovens, which creates an unhealthy atmosphere for adults, children and pets. For re-heating in your toaster oven, you'll need one or two Pyrex-type serving dishes, about a liter each. Heating leftovers for two or three people in a

toaster oven takes 15 minutes, not very much longer than a microwave.

6) Also use your toaster oven for breakfast. Take out some of the freezer vegetables you prepared, and sprinkle some cheese, such as mozzarella, provolone or parmesan over top, and heat it up for a healthy whole food breakfast, or break an egg over the vegetables. Neither of these will spike your insulin levels, unlike so many other dishes that we unfortunately have become accustomed to thinking of as breakfast foods.

7) Use your toaster oven to prepare hot, healthy lunches for yourself and your family. Invest in a good sized thermos with either glass or stainless steel (not aluminum) interior for each family member. While eating breakfast, heat up leftovers from last night, or a separately defrosted meal in your serving dish in the toaster oven, again for 10-15 minutes. Spoon it into each thermos. Then in each lunchbox, add a fork and little containers of nuts or some fresh fruit or some celery, cucumber, bell pepper or carrot sticks. You all will then have lunches that will be wonderfully nutritious, well balanced, and appetizing for every adult and child in your family. When all lunches are prepared together assembly-line style, the process will go faster than if each lunch is made separately. And your savings will begin to be obvious as your restaurant and fast food expenses plummet toward zero.

8) Take advantage of savings on seasonal produce. Get organic whenever possible. It has been by steadily rising consumer demand that growers have begun to get more and more organic produce into your local stores. Nature has no better gift than in-season organic berries. Here is a way to extend the seasonal savings. Fruit preserves can be

made unsweetened, and rely only on the natural sweetness of the fruit. Buy a case of about 4 pounds of berries when in season. Buy also 3 Granny Smith apples for pectin, which is a natural jelling agent. Peel and core the apples. Cut into about 1/2 –inch cubes. Place the apple pieces in a large pot, with about 3 pounds of washed and stemmed (if necessary) berries. (Keep the other one pound fresh for snacking.) Simmer the berries and apples on low for about an hour, while you are preparing your week's worth of meals. At the end of an hour, you should have a thin fruit spread. Take a potato masher and mash any remaining chunks of apple and berries as desired. Let it cool. The texture will get a little thicker. Freeze it in pint-size plastic containers. This makes a nice fruit spread which will keep indefinitely. A pleasant surprise is that the berry flavor is plenty sweet enough without added sweetener. Another food that will not spike your insulin. You can spread this with a nut butter on slices of apple or pear for breakfast or snacks.

9) Don't forget condiments. How often have you bought a bunch of parsley or cilantro with the good intention of using all of it, only to find most of it forgotten and wilted two weeks later, shoved behind other foods? When it's still fresh, chop it up finely and store in small plastic containers in the freezer. Then you can access it as needed for the one teaspoonful you may want, without having it wilt away before you get a chance to use it. But if you really want fresh herbs, grow them. My favorite Greek salad dressing calls for mint, oregano and parsley, which fortunately are all easy to grow, so I make sure I always have at least one plant of each growing, and I harvest sprigs each time I make the dressing. The fragrance alone of the just-picked herbs are what make the salad.

10) For the crockpot, food processor, thermoses and toaster oven recommended above, you may spend about $130. In order to recoup that investment, do yourself a huge favor, and change your mindset about potable liquids. There is really no good reason to drink anything other than water (R.O filtered or spring water). In fact, when we drink other liquids, we train ourselves to slake our thirst with different tastes than water, which then makes the taste of water seem strange. Since our bodies are 90% water, the only thing strange about this is our acquired perception of water as strange. Leave the heavy and expensive juices, teas, lattes and liquor at the store. Water is the only substance that can quench both the thirst we feel and the dehydration that almost everyone suffers to one degree or another. Drink it as you like it, with ice or without, with lemon or without, but reacquaint yourself with the one beverage that rehydrates and moisturizes all the way in to the cellular level and out to the skin: water.

When it comes to meal preparation, many people feel that their own lifestyle and difficult or hectic life circumstances keep them from attempting to cook. What is so beneficial about preparing your own whole, healthy food using some of the above steps is that any able-bodied adult can do it. Cooking big but freezing small is the best way for a single person to enjoy fully balanced home-cooked meals. For a busy parent with children of various ages, the kids can be recruited to help, and in turn receive the nutrients they most desperately need. Even toddlers can peel carrots, while older children can wash and chop foods. Some of our warmest childhood memories are from ordinary days and activities together with family members in the kitchen. Bestow the goodness on them too; pass the tradition to the next generation, so that cooking does not become just another lost art.

# Chapter 15
# Do you horrify others by abstaining from junk food?

Birthday parties, "The Holidays," Valentine's Day, Halloween and Thanksgiving: you cannot get very far along in the year before someone you know either thrusts a piece of cake or a box of donuts in front of you, or begs you to help them eat the huge quantity of baked goods they've made, or, in a gesture of niceness and inclusiveness offers you some sweets in an effort to initiate or reinforce friendship. In return you want to show your appreciation for their thoughts of you. The usual, unthinking way to do this is accept their treat and eat some together with them.

That is until you develop a habit, which becomes so routine that it is easier than accepting something that you know you'll regret later.

"Food sensitivities," you say. "Sugar actually makes me sick." (Dare yourself to say this. The first time you do, you'll wonder "what the heck am I saying?" And then you have to actually live up to the dare, and follow through with the conversation roughly as follows, or some variation thereof.)

"Are you diabetic?" is a common response.

"No, but any kind of sweeteners has always made me feel kind of sick. If I eat this now I will feel miserable tomorrow. But thank you so much anyway. I appreciate your thinking of me."

Your interlocutor may not be satisfied by your response and remind you of desserts that you have enjoyed together in the past.

"Every time I eat that stuff I feel terrible the next day. I'm not eating it anymore." (Say this last part with a touch of defiance. After all, you are at long last refusing to participate in this society's periodic mutual poisoning ritual. In fact, now that you have just taken this courageous stand, you will feel challenged and expected by others to maintain your position. And you will gradually begin to receive fewer and fewer offers of sweets.)

A persistent bearer of sweets might then respond, "Oh, but I made this myself with evaporated cane juice (or all-natural honey)."

"You made it yourself! No wonder it's so beautiful-looking. What a lot of work you must have done! I don't tolerate sweeteners though. Food sensitivity." This bit of redundancy almost always ends the persistent offer. But if you must continue, be prepared to do so. At this point, if you are feeling cheeky, you might even add "doctor's orders," since I am telling you to do this (unless of course you happen to be suffering a severe hypoglycemic episode at that moment). To really understand the devastating effect of any sweeteners on the body and mind, Dr. Mercola's book, Total Health [40] is an excellent primer on basic, sound nutritional guidelines.

Then if you're really feeling cheeky, you can turn the challenge around and ask: "Did you know there are 146 ways that sugar can ruin your health?" Dr. Nancy Appleton has gathered a large amount of such information from peer-reviewed medical journal articles and other medical literature. Her list of 146 ways is well worth reading, especially before a trip to a supermarket or restaurant.[41]

## Exchanging Carbs for Fats

People who eat refined carbohydrates or other processed foods often do not realize that when they crave a treat they would be more thoroughly satisfied by high-quality fat, not the carbs that they have always used to stifle the body's cries for fat. Nor do they realize that hunger is generally more completely satisfied by high-quality fat than by refined carbohydrates.

Why would we crave fat, when the processed food industry and medical profession have told us that it is bad for so long? Well this might have something to do with it: the brain is mostly made up of fat. As Dr. Walter Crinnion says, "We're all a bunch of fatheads!" The most desperately needed nutrient for growth and development of the brain from mid-pregnancy through infancy and childhood especially (but for adults also) is the omega-3 fatty acids found in fish oil and flax seed. For infants of course, the fat of breast milk is the most suitable, but that milk is greatly enriched by the mother's good nutrition and intake of omega-3 fatty acids.

---

[40] Mercola, Joseph, DO. Dr. Mercola's Total Health Program.
[41] Appleton, Nancy. PhD. "146 ways sugar ruins your health (with references)". Her famous article can be found on the internet at http://www.nancyappleton.com.

Anthropologists cite human intellectual and cultural development as having first blossomed in the vicinity of water and along waterways. Fish oil was an important part of the development of the human intellectual heritage. So were omega-6 fatty acids, which played a somewhat lesser but vital role. These are known as essential fatty acids because humans, omnivores that we naturally are, need to consume them.

Let's then consider some saturated fat treats that can be offered the next time you expect to be plied with refined carbs.

**Sashimi**

Sashimi is like sushi but without the rice. First, choose your fish very carefully for both freshness and quality. Wild Alaskan salmon is the high omega-3 fish that is known to be not as contaminated with mercury or PCBs as other fish. To be authentic, you can either use the 1/8$^{th}$ inch cut (sogi zukuri) or the 3/8$^{th}$ inch cut (hira zukuri). Cut across the grain through rectangular pieces of fish. A serving could be five or six pieces of the larger cut. Complement the fish with lemon slices, wasabi or horseradish, and shredded carrot and/or shredded cucumber.

**Cheese, apples, nuts**

Cheeses of various kinds should be more widely considered as snack food, fast food, appetizers, and elements of lunch boxes. Cheeses are now available in a variety of organic and/or raw forms. They complement nuts and/or chunks of apples, which in turn complement each other well for those whose lactose intolerance must omit the cheese.

**Chicken soup**

In cold weather, chicken soup is most highly prized for its soothing effect on upper respiratory infections. Naturopathic physician Kenneth Proefrock, NMD explains that the high amount of cysteine in chicken is a flatter molecule because of the sulfur group than most amino acids, which have globular-shaped carbon side chains. This results in respiratory secretions becoming more fluid and more easily slipping away from the nasopharyngeal membranes. I cook chicken in a crockpot with onion, celery and sea salt. If you are having a party or serving many people, the chicken soup can be ladled into coffee mugs. Just before serving, add minced garlic, chopped raw spinach or raw cilantro, and to give it a very tasty Chinese interpretation, toss in a tablespoon of sesame oil. These last ingredients can either make or break the flavor of chicken soup for many individuals, so you can leave them on the table for people to add as they please to the basic chicken soup that you give them.

# Chapter 16
# Whole Food Desserts

Why not just go out and have a cheesecake or ice cream? Why mix your healthy whole foods with something so naughty as desserts? Because it is not written anywhere that you have to punish your body when having a treat. If you eat desserts without sweeteners, then you can avoid the many chronic disease risks that come with sugar and its imitators, and still feel that you have eaten something sweet and filling.

The following recipes are for single servings of desserts, quite deliberately, for two reasons.

First, food that is made tends to get eaten, especially if it tastes good and doesn't have to be reheated. If you make a huge dessert, say a cake or pie for the whole family, they will end up ingesting more of this than would be prudent from the perspective of focusing most of one's diet on vegetables and proteins. When second and third helpings of dessert are available, you can be pretty sure they will get eaten, as everyone's better judgment and will power go out the window.

The second reason is that dessert is kind of like beer, wine or coffee. Children know it exists, but it could easily displace room for more nutrient dense vegetables and proteins in their small stomachs. If you have a whole fruit dessert while the kids are still awake, they may treat dinner as playtime, because they are saving room for fruit. The idea of dessert is that you must suffer through the vegetables and other healthy foods to get to your "just desserts." This programming, vegetables-bad, desserts-good, sets up associations in the mind that often never get broken, even into adulthood.

Because of this, children are best kept away from the idea of desserts altogether, even relatively healthy ones. Let the grown-ups enjoy a whole food dessert once in a great while after the kids are tucked in, and even then make it rare, because adults also need to keep their main food intake the highly nutrient dense vegetables and proteins.

So, to keep indulgence to a respectable minimum, and just as cocktail recipes are written for individual servings, we are listing the following desserts as single servings.

**Creamy Desserts**

For the following several desserts, we list real cream as a main ingredient. Ideally, you will be able to find raw cream, because it will provide the healthy enzymes and other proteins that have not been distorted by the flash pasteurization process used today. If you have access to raw goat or sheep milk, good for you! This is probably the best dairy available anywhere. If you do not have a goat share or other access to such dairy, you can also use cow milk. Cow dairy can be problematic for those not of Northern or

Western European ancestry. Goat proteins are considerably smaller, more easily absorbed and seem to be less allergenic for many people. If you can tolerate it, raw organic cow milk, as well as many other dairy products, including colostrum, is shipped throughout the U.S. by Organic Pastures in California. Their web address is http://www.organicpastures.com. Organic Pastures ships raw cream and other dairy products from their certified organic California dairy. You may also be able to find a local dairy farmer who may be persuaded to sell you raw dairy. Try the directory on the website of CSA Center, at http://www.csacenter.org, (part of Wilson College) to locate small family farms in your area. Sometimes "cow shares" for example at www.realmilk.com can be arranged for this purpose. Or you can use heavy cream or half and half, just so long as it is not ultra-pasteurized, because then its nutritional value is practically nothing. For adults and children who have trouble digesting dairy, many find that raw goat milk is digestible.

Then there are people who are horrified about eating real cream on fruits, but would think nothing about sprinkling sugar or artificial sweeteners over fruit. Their concerns are exactly the opposite of where they should be. For the many reasons given in Cholesterol Myths, by Uffe Ravnskov, MD, PhD and Nourishing Traditions, by Sally Fallon, the more fat in your milk the better. These books are both excellent nutritional resources and may be found online. And the more grass fed and pesticide-free the dairy cow or goat, the much better quality of fat you get, and the higher proportion of Omega 3 fatty acids available for brain health, artery health, heart health and joint and skin health. Most of the population studies have shown that it is possible to gorge yourself on dietary cholesterol and still keep the blood cholesterol very low. It is not only possible, but still practiced to this day by traditional cultures in various parts of the world. For a succinct and fascinating review of the medical debate on this subject, see also

Gary Taubes' article, entitled "What if it's all been a big fat lie?" at http://kanyak.com/fatlie.html

A lot of time when people reach for a candy bar or other sweet, they have been feeling a craving, and say something like, "I just feel I need a little *something* more, something sweet perhaps . . ." At these times, reaching for something sweet has become a conditioned habit, but it is definitely not those simple carbohydrates which make us feel completely satisfied and carry us through the ensuing hours. Rather, it is the fat in our diet that produces a sense of satisfaction and fullness after eating. The cream in the following recipes accomplishes that while complementing the flavors of the added fruits.

**Peaches and cream**

a peach, chopped in small chunks into a bowl
cream to partly cover

8 drops of almond extract
scant ¼ tsp vanilla extract

Sally Fallon combines almond extract with peaches for a nice flavor combination. Here we add raw cream for nutritional balance, and vanilla to make it incredibly good tasting. Stir well to mix in the strongly flavored extracts.

**Dates and pecans**

1 or 2 dates
1/3 cup pecans
cream to partly cover

Pit and chop dates into small pieces. Add pecans and stir till date pieces are well distributed. Add cream.

**Chocolate and banana**

Approx 1" x 2" rectangle of unsweetened dark chocolate
A banana

In the baking section of the supermarket you'll find unsweetened chocolate for baking. (Okay, so it's not exactly whole food, but at least it doesn't have added sweeteners or synthetics, and it's as close as we temperate clime folks can get to the cacao pods.) Ghirardelli's is the most convenient for this, but any kind of unsweetened "baking chocolate" will do. Simply alternate bites of the chocolate with bites of banana, pear or another not-too-acidic fruit. That's it; just alternate bites to balance flavors.

**Chocolate almond pudding**

This is a really fast way to satisfy a sweet tooth and keep you away from health-destroying junk.

2 tablespoons almond butter or peanut butter
1 teaspoon unsweetened chocolate powder
1 teaspoon carob powder
3 tablespoons raw milk or almond milk (optional)

Stir together for a few moments till smooth. None of the amounts need be exact. The chocolate will satisfy that craving, while the carob sweetens it up enough, and the nut butter provides good texture, as well as an Omega-6 fat background to satisfy the appetite. The milk thins it, but that can be minimized if you don't mind a very thick consistency.

**Chocolate from Marz**

a frozen banana (first peeled and cut into chunks)
a 1-2" square of unsweetened (baking) chocolate
nutmeg, dash
1/4 teaspoon vanilla
1 tablespoon flaxseeds
2 tablespoons walnuts
2 tablespoons water

Naturopathic physician Russell Marz, ND agreed to share this recipe with us, which is especially helpful for the high quality omega-3 fatty acids contained in the flax and walnuts as well as the antioxidants that have been found in chocolate. Mix all ingredients in a high-powered blender till consistent. This dessert has a chunky ice cream-like texture. For birthday celebrations it would make a good substitute for cake and ice cream.

**Carob and cream**

I like to take about 3 tablespoons of raw organic cream. Raw milk will also do. Add 2 scoops of probiotic flora, such as Primal Defense and a quarter to a half-teaspoon of carob powder. Carob powder is the ground, dried carob pod. The carob tree is of Mediterranean origin and also grows in the Americas. If constipation is an issue, use moderation with carob powder, as large quantities can have a constipating effect. Stir well. No sweetener is needed for this creamy, delightful treat, which is thick enough to be eaten as a pudding. It thickens as it is left standing. Almond milk may be used by those who are lactose intolerant for a different consistency but somewhat similar flavor.

**Simplest recipe of all: whole fruit popsicles**

Peaches, plums, nectarines, watermelon, berries, honeydew or cantaloupe
(Or a colorful combination of these)
Popsicle molds

Don't forget about the kids altogether. The whole fruit that you may give them for a snack is all the yummier on a summer afternoon when frozen on a popsicle stick. Any of the above fruits works quite well. Cut the fruit into small chunks, and stuff them into popsicle molds. Kids enjoy making their own popsicles, so let even the little ones do this job. Just make sure you pack the fruit in tight, minimizing air pockets. Watermelon probably works the best, but all of the above fruits are great for this too. Freeze for a few hours at least.

* * *

The whole foods mentioned in this book do not elicit an insulin spike as do concentrated fruit and fruit juice, because they have all the fiber of the whole food to slow the entry of natural sugars to the bloodstream. The real damage of typical sugared desserts is to elevate your insulin, which itself is certain high risk for heart disease and atherosclerosis.

In contrast, when the bounties of nature take the shortest path from the earth to your mouth, that is, not passing through a food processing plant in an industrial park before they get to you, then you are giving your body what humans have needed for countless generations. Let your occasional dessert indulgence be as natural and compatible with your body as the rest of your food. If you put whole foods together right, they can be quite delicious, and not upset your optimal biochemical balance.

# Chapter 17
# Hot chocolate with no sugar, no synthetics

In the winter, hot chocolate is a great temptation. Here's how to make it without sugar (hence without glucose and insulin whipsawing) and as close to whole foods as we can get you at this time, *and* still have it taste recognizably hot, liquid and chocolaty.

You will need:

½ tsp powdered licorice root

(If a local health food store does not have this, you may have to get it online. Only the powdered licorice root is fine enough and makes a thick enough liquid to work nicely.)

1 x 1-inch square unsweetened (baking) chocolate
Ghirardelli's works best because it is so thin. Or you may be able to find unsweetened powdered plain cocoa at your store.

Cream or milk to taste

For one cup of hot chocolate, heat drinking water to boil. Pour water into coffee mug over licorice root powder and chocolate. If you use solid chocolate, you will have to stir a bit to break it up and disperse it, and even then it won't completely dissolve, but will work well enough. Powdered unsweetened cocoa powder will dissolve easily. If you like cream, leave room for it at the top and add to taste.

Licorice root is one of the botanical medicines most frequently used by naturopathic physicians and herbalists. It is the most nourishing plant known for the adrenal glands. The adrenals are a part of the body that are heavily damaged and depleted by accumulated mental and emotional stress over the years. By middle age, many people's adrenal glands are functioning at low levels. Licorice is also nourishing for the liver and has been used to soothe stomach ulcers.

Licorice root is also anti-oxidant and anti-viral, two wonderful properties for fighting viral infections this time of year. Licorice is also demulcent and anti-spasmodic, specifically for coughs, and it can be used in the above form to relieve coughs.

Licorice boosts the immune system, which is quite the opposite of the effect of conventional hot chocolate. The conventional variety contains sugar, which inactivates your white blood cells, your immune system's cold and flu fighters, for a period of five to 24 hours – not quite what we need this time of year. Especially with the hardest part of the flu season ahead of us.

Just watch out for a slight stimulant effect of the chocolate if you are not used to it. Chocolate contains theobromine, which is chemically similar to theophylline in caffeine. In fact, if you choose to leave out the chocolate altogether and just have the licorice, you will still have a warm and pleasing beverage.

Also, it is possible for someone with high blood pressure to have an increase with licorice, if consumed regularly. But if your blood pressure is within a reasonable range, one cup should be fine. Consult with your naturopathic physician if this is a concern for you.

**Hot licorice for cold and flu season**

1 teaspoon powdered licorice
1 rounded teaspoon L-glutamine powder
½ tsp glycine powder
1 teaspoon larch arabinogalactans

This potent brew is especially helpful for fighting off respiratory infections. We begin with the anti-viral, cough-soothing and immune enhancing effects of licorice. Then we add L-glutamine, the most common amino acid in food, one that can be taken at 1-2 rounded teaspoons per day, with no ill effect that I have observed in adults or children. Glutamine is also immune-enhancing as well as necessary mucous-membrane rebuilding material. Without it, the damage to membranes of the pharynx, larynx and GI tract following a cold can last for weeks. Glutamine greatly shortens the healing and rebuilding process. Larch is immune-enhancing and specifically important for increasing T1 cells, an important advantage to have in fighting off respiratory illness.

# Chapter 18
# Dietary fat: A benevolent villain

Non-fat and fat-free and low-fat foods have become so aggressively marketed for so long to the American public that it's enough to make the average person stop in surprise at the reminder that a full 20 to 30% of our calories should come from fat, in a well-balanced diet, according to consensus within a certain margin, which is rare, among most food experts (nutritionists, dieticians, naturopathic physicians, etc.). You may look with disgust at the gristle on meat, or at a well-buttered piece of toast, assuming as many do that dietary fat must be similar to, or causative of, body fat, because of use of the same word.

What most people don't know is that the pathways of metabolism, (meaning food breakdown and transformation) that are the same in everybody's body, take fat through a common breakdown cycle with sugars and starches, circulating through a process known as the citric acid cycle or Krebs cycle. If you haven't had organic chemistry, the Krebs cycle is a huge can of worms that you may not want to want to learn about right now. But one important take home point is this: If you have a high-fat diet, your body reduces its manufacture of fatty acids, meaning that it's reducing the building blocks of your body fat. On the other hand, high carb diets, including fat-free diets cause an increase in enzyme synthesis, which increases fatty acid synthesis, which means your body is then making more of those building blocks of bodily fat. In other words, a high fat diet gives rise to less body fat. A low-fat diet gives rise to more body fat. Our ancestors ate lard and way more butter than we do, and were thin. We got rid of lard entirely and go easy on the butter, and we are much heavier. Why does it work this way? Because your body wants a consistent level of fat in the liver and will adjust its own manufacture accordingly to keep things at a consistent level. Stop eating fat, and you make more fat. Continue eating fat, and you don't need to make as much.

Another good thing about dietary fat has recently been discovered by researchers at the Ohio State University Comprehensive Cancer Center. We always knew that fat soluble vitamins, such as A, D, E and K, as well as wax-based nutrients, such as Co Q10 are absorbed best with some fat. What we did not know, which the research uncovered, was that the carotenoids, which are important cancer-fighting nutrients, are absorbed 2 to 18 times better with a high fat food than a non-fat food. Eating fat in the same meal was found to be sufficient for the optimal absorption of fat. For example, if the meal includes a meat (saturated fat), then the carotenoids from generally warm-colored vegetables in the meal will be absorbed.

In a different study in Germany, it was found that trans-fats, such as hydrogenated oils, made the absorption of fat-soluble vitamins even worse than if no fat was eaten. So the quality of fats certainly matters. Omega-3 fats are the most generally useful and the hardest to get enough of in your diet. Remember that the best sources for these are wild salmon, sardines, herring, anchovies, flax seed and walnuts. Also important are the Omega-6 fatty acids found in borage and evening primrose oils, such as the combination of oils in Udo's Oil, available in health food stores.

# Chapter 19
# How to cut, store and eat organic beef without breaking your budget

Just trying to imagine the price of organic beef can inspire sticker shock in consumers. However, there is a way to have your beef and not pay a fortune.

If you have a nearby health food supermarket that sells organic beef, you may be able to find eye round, bottom round or London broil for about $6.00 to $9.00 per pound. Organic grass–fed beef was only available from New Zealand for a time, but more and more is being raised in the U.S.

Ask the butcher to slice the round in ¾" to 1" thick slices. When you get home, put each slice in a separate zip-type plastic bag and freeze them. This way, you can defrost one steak at a time, per person, for sautéing or grilling. Then each steak ends up costing just a little over a dollar.

### But if you don't live near such a store...

If on the other hand you don't have a local source of organic beef, there are two other options.

Grassland Beef sells a bottom round roast. Their website is: www.grasslandbeef.com

### Heirloom beef

Another option is beef from heirloom breeds of cattle, such as Hereford, Devon, Highlander and Galloway. You may find a farmer near you raising this cattle, but if not, you can have huge cuts of this beef shipped from Lobels in New York. They are online at: www.lobels.com. Heirloom cattle are grass-fed and raised on small family farms using traditional methods. Raised without hormones, pesticides or subtherapeutic antibiotics, this kind of beef is comparable to organic beef. Furthermore, because it is grass-fed, it is high in the omega-3 fatty acids, which are so necessary for good brain, skin, immune and heart health.

# Chapter 20
# Food as Medicine: We eat our way into our symptoms, and we can eat our way back out

***"Let food be your medicine and medicine be your food."*** **- Hippocrates**

We live at a strange crossroads in history. Over the last several decades, the human species has been hypnotized by the temptations offered by the chemical and pharmaceutical industries. The 1950's ushered in the "better living through chemicals" age. And we believed, and we bought and swallowed and injected and are still consuming them in massive amounts, and, most recklessly, injecting such chemicals as ethyl mercury, ethylene glycol (antifreeze), aluminum and formaldehyde into our babies as part of vaccines, without any prior safety testing.

But now with massive chronic disease plaguing our most industrialized populations, autism closely following children's shots, (by parents' documentation, in defiance of the pronouncements of safety by the drug industry) and more pathology coincident with concentrated chemicals, we are beginning to wake up from our long post-World War II slumber. Now begins the next era when synthetic chemicals are starting to be seen as, however useful in many applications, best kept at a distance from our bodies, our homes, public spaces and wilderness.

The old era of unthinking reliance on a synthetic existence is showing severe disadvantages, just as the urgency to forge new relationships with nature is becoming apparent. Plants and other whole foods are coming into their own new era as naturopathic physicians and other well-informed health practitioners rely on them for their central role in healing. Within our lifetimes, whole food will eclipse pharmaceuticals in medical practice, as the general public awakens to its far superior healing capacity. But the allopathic profession will be the slowest to catch on, just as most physicians of the early 20$^{th}$ century refused to believe that absence of certain nutrients could bring on such horrible diseases as scurvy, pellagra and beriberi. Then as now, allopaths were eager to lay blame for these diseases on microbes, until . . . oops! limes cured the "limey" British sailors of their scurvy, and we saw that Vitamin B3 prevented pellagra, while Vitamin B1 prevented beriberi and Vitamin D prevented rickets. As usual, allopathy corrects itself long after the natural physicians are already healing patients. In fact, evidence now shows that even bubonic plague, which allopathy still attributes to bacteria known as *Yersinia pestis*, was more likely to strike those with low Vitamin C intakes.

But what would possess a person to think that food could possibly be medicine? Our first clue is the structure of our intestines. Whatever comes into the mouth later travels through miles of efficient tubing that extracts certain molecules from the food we eat, then converts them to one common molecule, Acetyl Co-A, from which the building blocks of the body are then made: protein, glucose and (healthy-type) fats. The intestines are great little machines, but not omnipotent. That is, they can convert food molecules to Acetyl Co-A, because food has familiar and malleable combinations of carbon, hydrogen, oxygen and nitrogen. But it cannot do that with bizarre substances that the body is unfamiliar with, such as petrochemical products and synthetic substances used in pharmaceuticals. The body has no experience with many of these substances, has little clue what to do with them, and often excretes them, which may explain why placebos so often equal or surpass drugs in clinical trials. More often, though, as the body tries to either detoxify or wall off the offending invader drug, it creates new metabolites, which have multiple pharmaceutical effects, some of which may be quite harmful.

Food, on the other hand, is right at home in the body, since our species (like the others) has always processed it, and we have become quite efficient eating machines as a result. Therefore, we easily break down ingested protein to its component amino acids. These then in turn get rearranged into the proteins that our genes tell us to make, all of the busy construction that takes place in the womb, and for the rest of us: replacement of lost skin and membrane cells, slightly longer fingernails, hair, scabs over wounds, etc. Carbohydrates and dietary fat get broken down to Acetyl Co-A and rearranged to form the molecules our body needs to function, because this is how our bodies have been handling things for all of our existence as a species. How would the body be able to do that from a pharmaceutical? It can't. It's like trying to make your car run on orange juice.

Except for the last century in industrialized society, both humans and animals have almost exclusively relied on plants for their medicine. In fact, it is instructive that, as wild animals are still known to seek plants that are appropriate treatments for whatever illness may be present, rather than also having access to our pharmaceuticals, animals observed in the wild are still free of chronic disease, even when living all the way to their maximum lifespan. Our veterinary and zoo populations, on the other hand, present a very different picture: cancers, constipation and pancreatitis are seen quite commonly among people's well-loved pets who are subject to a highly processed diet as well as synthetic pharmaceuticals by us, their well-intentioned owners and the pet food industry.

Whether we were created or evolved, we have been so intimately connected to plants for all of our existence as a species that we cannot live without them. We connect with plants and exchange with plants down to our very cells and our smallest molecules. That is why they heal us like nothing else can. Our historical reliance on plants has been an integral part of every human society. Plants and humans resonate on levels that are still beyond our comprehension, including biochemical and physiological levels, and some would say aesthetic and emotional as well. How could humans and plants so closely have shared this earth, one with the other, and not had complementary, multi-faceted relationships with each other? Hippocrates said, "Let your food be your medicine and your medicine be your food." Medicine is what you get when the most appropriate plant is given to an ill person. The plant kingdom does play the major role of all foods in this wonderfully beneficial relationship for us.

### Why do herbs have multiple properties, if pharmaceuticals only do one thing?

Pharmaceuticals are highly refined homogeneous substances. The molecules contained in drugs are strictly selected for very specific effects on the body and are mostly synthetic. Only about 25% of pharmaceuticals are derived from plants. The rest are mostly chemically derived from tightly controlled chemical reactions.

Whole plants, on the other hand, particularly wild ones, such as are commonly used in herbal medicine have hundreds, sometimes thousands of chemical constituents. Such wild plants as chamomile, plantain, creosote bush and dandelion are medicinal herbs of longstanding use, especially for gastric ulcer and infant colic, cough and interstitial cystitis, antioxidant and joint inflammation, and edema and gallbladder sluggishness respectively. They have a long history of adaptation to various climates and soils, and they have a wide range. As such, they have developed many defenses against their natural enemies. These numerous chemical constituents in turn comprise multiple therapeutic uses, as well as a resonance with our bodies, mostly because our ancestors for countless millenia frequently consumed such foods and left us with the kind of metabolism that actually works very well with these plants. After ingestion of a plant, the various plant constituents come together in a synergy of its parts, in such a way that one part that may be toxic on its own is modulated by the presence of the other plant constituents. Because our bodies have been adapted to these plants as foods, they are much more compatible with good health than synthetic chemicals are.

**Quality whole foods are the currency of life**

Whether you believe in creation, or evolution or are undecided, most of us would agree that our bodies (that is our anatomy and biochemistry, our metabolism of food) is substantially the same as that of our recent ancestors. What happens when we substitute factory chemicals such as synthetic food and pharmaceuticals for the water and many different nutrients that our cells and our children's cells and internal organs need simply to function well? In fact, the very sad consequences of the latest generations' food and medication choices is becoming more apparent everyday as we are now seeing chronic diseases such as diabetes and heart disease become epidemic in our society. The United States has the worst health status (life expectancy and infant mortality) of any of the industrialized nations, yet we spend the most money on healthcare and take the most pharmaceuticals. Why are Americans getting sicker and sicker while drugging ourselves more and more?

**Forget what you ate until today. What you eat from now on is vitally important to your continued well-being.**

Until just a few generations ago, our ancestors were wonderfully fit and healthy compared with present-day generations. The majority lived good, active, healthy lives and ultimately died peacefully in their sleep. Today that is a rarity. Whereas chronic disease, chronic pain, and prolonged end-of-life care were practically unheard of for our ancestors, it is becoming much more the expected outcome for us. What single difference between these two centuries impacts our bodies the strongest? The overwhelmingly different factor in our lives is the refined, processed, chemical products that we eat, that our ancestors simply did not eat. If our species, for better or worse, whether created, evolved or in-between, performs best on whole foods (vegetables, fruits, meats, etc.), then we can understand that putting synthetic liquid or solid wastes in the body will simply trash our most valuable possession: our own good health.

## Food Solutions for Medical Problems

When it comes to medical problems most people tend to think of hospitals, doctor's offices, prescriptions for drugs. However, naturopathic physicians have found that the most effective tools of healing are the food that you eat. If it is true that "you are what you eat," and that your body's cells entirely turn over every few months, then what you will be and how you will feel a few months from now has *everything* to do with what you eat and what you don't eat between now and that time.

Indeed, naturopathic physicians find that it takes people even less than that amount of time to start feeling wonderful. From babies to senior citizens, people who start eating better feel way better beginning on the first or second day, with dramatic improvements still over the first few weeks, and maintained wellbeing after that. Cravings for unhealthy food *can be eliminated*, and your ND can help you with that. There are people who live in states that don't license naturopathic physicians who fly great distances so that they can see a naturopathic physician who helped them in the past, or to bring in their loved ones for naturopathic treatment.

Many Americans believe that illness or pain is so strong that it must be slammed down with a strong drug. It would amaze most people to know that naturopathic physicians get far more complete and permanent results with their patients by convincing them to improve what they eat, and by creating together with the patient an eating plan that the patient is willing to try. The night-and-day difference of good food vs. bad food is really not so amazing when you consider that the molecules of whole healthy food are so much more similar to the molecules of our own bodies than are drugs. This is why they heal us like nothing else can.

# Chapter 21
# Organic food: not just for white people

LaDonna Redmond got her business inspiration in her own neighborhood of Austin, on Chicago's West Side. She noticed that you could buy all sorts of items there, but could not find even an organic tomato. "Folks say black people won't eat organic food – that all we want to eat is Cheetos," she says. Such ridiculous stereotyping keeps marketing and distribution of organic and other healthy foods away from black communities.

So Redmond decided to correct the problem herself. She launched a farmer's market in her inner-city neighborhood to bring in fresh organic produce. Having only one supermarket and dozens of fast food and processed food outlets serving 117,000 residents, there was plenty of room for a better source of food in

Austin. "We need to get folks the information to make a choice," she says. "Eating is a political act."

Now on Saturdays during the summer an elementary school playground becomes the scene of stands selling okra, collards, turnips and other produce grown by African-American farmers in Kankakee County, south of Chicago. The Redmond family also started growing vegetables in their own backyard, which has now expanded to a working farm on six vacant lots. Last year they grew 40,000 pounds of produce.

As a result, five Chicago universities have teamed up with Redmond's non-profit group, the Institute for Community Resource Development, under a grant from the W.K. Kellogg Foundation to study the food needs of the Austin community. They have already begun salad bars and nutrition classes in neighborhood schools, and plans are underway to build a food co-op. The Austin Farmers Market thrives now over a decade old, and Redmond has been named a Food Innovator by Time Magazine.

# Chapter 22
# Can you afford NOT to eat whole, organic foods? A price comparison

A common perception is that whole organic food is so expensive that it is out-of-budget for the average family or even for the average single consumer. It is also commonly perceived that the average grocery purchase of processed foods at a neighborhood supermarket, using the store discounts, makes the processed food diet within the budget of most families.

**If you go along with those who accept the above hypothesis on faith, you may be quite surprised by what you find in this chapter.**

Knowing what I spend on groceries in an average week for my all whole food, mostly organic-eating family, I had to test the conventional wisdom for myself. So one day I went to a typical supermarket right around the corner from me to see how the other half lives . . .

**Health nut stalks supermarket aisles with notebook in hand**

Jotting down in my notebook many processed foods as well as their weights and prices, with all the store savings, I prepared a long list of foods from which I could construct a hypothetical week's worth of processed food for a family of three. Below you will find a menu of all processed food items for a week, and a list of prices for all the groceries that I hypothetically bought. Then I assembled my hypothetical purchases into a meal plan for a family of three, which you will see below, along with the price list.

Following that, you will find a week's menu and price list for mostly organic, all whole food meals for the same family of three.

**Ground rules**

For the sake of simplicity and realistic comparison, I stuck to the following constraints:

- There are no leftovers from before the beginning of the week, nor saved at the end (empty refrigerator beginning and end, and no throwing out food; everything purchased gets eaten by the three hypothetical family members).
- Unless specified otherwise, all beverage consumption is water.
- There are no separate snacks, except for Sunday afternoon, unless an individual saves part of a meal to snack on later.

- Neither the cheapest generic brands, nor the most expensive brands were chosen, but rather a brand in the middle, especially if it was on sale.
- Portions are listed per family member of a three-person family, although the heartiest appetite in the family may consume some part of the portion left by the smallest appetite. It is assumed that everyone eats the same food at the same time everyday, and that the six ounces of soda at every lunch is either carried in a thermos to work or school, or that this family is on vacation at home, eating every meal at home together and pouring their soda directly from a large bottle kept in the refrigerator.
- It is assumed that no family member is deliberately restricting calories, or is otherwise restricting any type of food.

The cold bottled coffee at breakfast may seem a bit extravagant, but consider that this replaces visits to coffee shops or any other form of coffee or tea or recreational beverage. Also, the all-processed food family does not get milk with their cereal, but rather cold, bottled, sugared coffee, just to keep everything processed, for the sake of a truer comparison.

**The processed food menu, per person, for one week**

<u>Sunday:</u>

B: 3 pancakes with syrup
7.5 oz. cold bottled coffee
L: 13 oz. canned ravioli
6 oz soda
Sn: ice cream sandwich
D: 3.5 oz. frozen breaded fish
4 oz salad with dressing
6 oz soda
ice cream bar

**Monday:**
B: 4 oz. bagel with 5 oz. jelly
L: 9 oz frozen lunch
6 oz. soda
D: 8 oz ground beef patties with ketchup, relish
6 oz french fries
ice cream bar

**Tuesday:**
B: 3 oz. sugared cereal
7.5 oz. cold bottled coffee instead of milk
L: 3.5 oz. frozen breaded fish
6 oz soda
D: 7 oz frozen corn dogs
2 oz frozen potato pancakes
ketchup, relish
ice cream bar

**Wednesday:**
B: 2 toaster pastries
7.5 oz. cold bottled coffee
L: 9 oz frozen lunch
6 oz soda
D: frozen TV dinner, individual
1 serving flavored rice
ice cream bar

**Thursday:**
B: 2 toaster pastries
7.5 oz. cold bottled coffee
L: 9 oz frozen lunch
6 oz soda
D: 8 oz lb frozen ground beef patties with ketchup, relish
6 oz frozen french fries

ice cream sandwich

**Friday:**

B: 3 oz. sugared cereal
7.5 cold bottled coffee
L: 9 oz frozen lunch
6 oz soda
D: 7 oz corn dogs
2 oz potato pancakes
ketchup
relish
ice cream sandwich

**Saturday:**

B: 3 pancakes with syrup
L: 9 oz frozen pizza
6 oz soda
D: 6 oz frozen pork chops with gravy
1 serving macaroni and cheese
6 oz soda
ice cream sandwich

**The price list for the processed food menu:**[42]

| | | |
|---|---|---|
| 17 oz | pork chops with gravy | $6.99 |
| 3 lbs | ground beef patties | $8.99 |
| 13 oz | potato pancakes | $4.19 |
| 2 lbs | frozen french fries | $2.79 |
| 2.67 lbs | corn dogs | $5.99 |
| 27 oz | frozen pizza | $4.99 |
| 12 | ice cream bars | $2.99 |
| 12 | ice cream sandwiches | $2.99 |
| 6 | toaster pastries | $2.00 |

[42] Amounts reflect prices in effect in 2005.

| | | |
|---|---|---|
| 6 | frozen pastries | $2.00 |
| 16 oz. | small jar of jelly | $1.99 |
| 12 oz. | bagels | $0.99 |
| 1 lb | TV dinner | $3.89 |
| 1 lb | TV dinner | $3.89 |
| 14.5 oz | TV dinner | $2.50 |
| 21 oz. | fillets frozen breaded fish | $5.79 |
| 68 oz | soda | $0.99 |
| 6 pk 16.9 oz | soda | $2.99 |
| 40 oz | canned ravioli | $2.99 |
| 1 bottle | ketchup | $0.99 |
| 1 bottle | relish | $0.99 |
| 1 sm bot. | salad dressing | $1.99 |
| 17 oz | sugared cereal | $3.89 |
| 12 | bottles of cold coffee with cream | $13.47 |
| 1 sm bot. | syrup | $1.50 |
| 20 pancakes | pancake mix - add only water | $2.39 |
| 3 svgs | flavored rice | $1.49 |
| 12 oz | packaged salad | $2.99 |
| 12 oz | frozen lunches | $24.00 |
| | | **$123.64** |

* * *

**How does whole food compare?**

Now consider a menu prepared entirely from whole organic and free-range foods. One might consider such a diet to be extravagantly expensive. Yet the cost for a week's worth of organic whole food groceries for a family of three is about the same as for the "cheap" processed food.

The same rules apply as with the processed food. No leftovers from the beginning of the week or saved at the end (empty refrigerator beginning and end, with no waste). No restaurant eating or take-out. No beverages other than water. No snacks except for what one person may save for later from his/her apportioned meal. No deliberate calorie restriction, and everyone eats till full.

All meals are listed for one person only of a 3-person family, assuming that those with larger appetites may have more, and those of smaller appetites may have an equal amount less, in order to balance out to the average portions listed below.

A significant difference is that the processed food eating family gets a dessert of an ice cream bar, while the whole food eating family gets no dessert. The whole food eating family however generally gets much bigger meal portions. The reason behind this is partly demographic realism: those who eat denatured food are missing nutrients that they seek in desserts and other denatured foods, whereas whole food eaters feel completely full when eating in proper proportions for their metabolic types. See chapter on metabolic types.

**The whole organic foods menu, per person, for one week**

A typical week's menu at our house would look like the following: Only the sliced bacon, sliced cheeses, cream cheese and goat milk are pre-packaged. Every dish is prepared at home from scratch.

**<u>Sunday</u>**
B: 2 eggs cooked in butter
2 slices bacon
L: salad: spinach, romaine, bell pepper, 2 oz. muenster cheese, cilantro, sea salt, olive oil
Sn: 8 oz. apple

D: 16 oz. chicken stew: part of whole chicken with potatoes, onions, celery, carrots, olive oil, balsamic vinegar, water, sea salt and curry powder

**Monday**

B: 12 oz. apple slices with 2 oz. almond butter
L: 16 oz. left over chicken stew
5 oz. orange
1 oz. pumpkin seeds
D: 8 oz. curry: eggplant, potato, onion, bell pepper, butter, curry powder, salt

**Tuesday:**

B: smoothie: 10 oz. goat milk and one banana and 3 oz. raspberries
L: 16 oz. leftover chicken stew
2 oz. cashews
2 oz. carrots
D: 3 oz. salmon with ground dill
Salad: spinach, romaine, 1 oz. muenster cheese, cilantro, salt, olive oil

**Wednesday:**

B: 12 oz apple slices with 1 oz. cream cheese
L: 8 oz. left over eggplant curry
2 oz. Cheddar cheese
1 oz. pumpkin seeds
D: 4 oz. acorn squash
5 oz. Broccoli raab sauteed in olive oil

**Thursday:**

B: smoothie: 10 oz. goat milk, 3 oz. raspberries and one banana

L: 2 oz. leftover salmon, 4 oz. acorn squash and 5 oz. broccoli raab
3 oz. cashews
D: 16 oz. crockpot roast: beef, potatoes, celery, onions, carrots, sea salt

**Friday:**
B: 12 oz. apple slices with 2 oz. almond butter
L: 8 oz. leftover eggplant curry
2 oz. Cheddar cheese
2 oz. carrots
D: 16 oz. leftover roast beef stew

**Saturday:**
B: 2 eggs with 1 oz. cream cheese and spinach, cooked in butter
2 slices bacon
L: 16 oz. leftover roast beef stew
5 oz. orange
D: salad: sardines, romaine, 1 oz. muenster cheese, cilantro, salt, olive oil

**The price list for the whole organic food menu:**[43]

| | | |
|---|---|---|
| 1.88 lbs. | organic oranges | $1.86 |
| 8.27 lbs. | organic Fuji apples | 12.32 |
| 3.23 lbs | organic bananas | 2.87 |
| 2.47 lbs. | organic potatoes | 1.95 |
| 2.65 lbs | * organic onions | 3.42 |
| 1 lb. | organic baby carrots | 1.39 |
| 1.91 lbs | * organic acorn squash | 2.46 |

[43] Amounts reflect 2005 typical prices.

| | | |
|---|---|---|
| one | organic bell pepper | 1.05 |
| 1.4 lbs | * organic eggplant | 2.79 |
| 1 bunch | * organic cilantro | 0.99 |
| 2 bunches | * organic broccoli raab | 4.08 |
| 1 bunch | organic spinach | 1.99 |
| 1 head | organic romaine | 1.39 |
| 1 lb. | raw cashews | 4.29 |
| 6 oz. | * pumpkin seeds | 1.54 |
| 12 oz | almond butter, fresh ground | 5.25 |
| one whole | organic free-range chicken | 9.79 |
| 1 lb. | copper river salmon | 12.99 |
| 2.25 lbs. | organic free range chuck roast beef | 11.23 |
| one package | no hormone bacon | 3.49 |
| 1/2 gal | goat milk | 4.78 |
| 1/2 lb | organic butter | 1.79 |
| 1 dozen | organic free range eggs | 3.49 |
| 8 oz | no hormone cream cheese | 2.29 |
| 12 oz | sliced muenster cheese | 3.99 |
| 12 oz | sliced cheddar cheese | 3.99 |
| 20 oz. | frozen raspberries | 3.18 |
| 1 can | sardines | 1.79 |
| 1/2 pint | organic olive oil | 4.99 |
| 2 oz | sea salt | 0.20 |
| 1 oz | curry powder | 0.34 |
| 1 oz | dill powder | 0.17 |
| small bottle | balsamic vinegar | 2.99 |
| | | **$121.13** |

We made no attempt to quantify the salad ingredients. Fresh plants and salads are such an anarchy of ingredients, they defy standardization. Cooking large meals with whole foods is a little trickier to quantify than packages of pre-weighed processed foods.

The difference is made up in the leftovers. For example, the large crockpot chicken stew at the beginning of the week, the eggplant curry in the middle of the week, and the roast beef at the end are massive enough not only for everyone's dinner, but also for two days' lunches as well, with generous one-pound portions. The one-pound portions of stew are about half added water by weight.

Both the salmon dinners and squash-and-broccoli raab dinners are small enough that the leftovers put together make just one lunch for the family. The advantage to cooking enormous crockpot or Dutch oven meals, with subsequent leftovers, is that although it is more time-consuming to prepare whole food from scratch, it is easier just to do it in fewer larger amounts during the week. If this still seems daunting, please see the chapter, "Cook Whole Food from Scratch, and Keep Your Day Job."

### The bottom line

You will notice the savings of $2.51 with a mostly organic whole food diet In fact, our organic food price list shows higher than realistic prices in two ways: The prices shown are at retail health food stores in the Phoenix area. But also in this area, there are at least three organic food-buying groups, with prices for organic produce at about $1.30 to $1.50 per pound. To find organic food buying groups, co-ops, health food stores, local retail farms and farmers markets in your area, see www.localharvest.org.

Furthermore, if you have a backyard, especially here in the Southwest, you can save further in ways that processed food eaters can't: Almost all year we grow salad greens, herbs, braising greens of some kind and/or various squashes. The salad herbs oregano, thyme, rosemary, mint and parsley never quit here in any season! In colder climates and in apartments, these herbs may be grown in containers near a sunny window. Subtracting the prices of what we are currently pulling out of our back yard garden from what is on the sample menu:

| | |
|---|---|
| Organic cilantro: | $0.99 |
| And organic broccoli raab: | $4.08 |
| We save an additional | $5.07 |

Which means we spend only $121.13 - $5.07 = $116.06 in an average week for a 3-person family, which is $7.58 less than the family eating all processed food. Of course, gardeners in colder climates tend to have really prolific harvests in summer and fall, which is when they will realize much better savings. Processed food eaters are entirely dependent on commercial supply, no matter what the season.

However, the biggest savings of the whole-food eating family has yet to be calculated, as we consider the difference in medical care needs between whole food eaters on the one hand, and those who will continue eating for decades such chemicals as MSG (aka hydrolyzed wheat protein and several other names), carcinogens or nerve poisons (a.k.a. pesticides and aspartame), sugar and other sweeteners, as well as margarine and other trans-fatty acids, to name some of the most infamous processed food ingredients. As a wise saying goes, the best reason to eat organic is that pesticides don't know when to stop killing.

**Moment of truth**

Now answer honestly: can you afford NOT to eat whole organic food?

# Chapter 23
# Trick yourself into drinking more water

How many times a year to you get browbeaten about not drinking enough water? Worst part is, those dreary scolds are right. You get so busy you don't get around to drinking your eight to ten glasses of water a day.

Here's how you can trick yourself into drinking more water. Spike it with substantial lemon. This means not just the little lemon slice floating on top of the glass like you get in restaurants. It means cutting a good size 3 inch by 1 inch wedge of fresh lemon, squeezing it into your water, then throwing the rind in your water for good measure.

The way it works is the lemon is not only sour, but also astringent. This has a slight drying effect on the tongue. So the tongue, that same spoiled brat that has been known to demand unhealthy food, now feels dry, and demands . . . more water!

Diluting the juice of a hefty lemon wedge in a 16-ounce glass of water is enough to produce the drying effect necessary to motivate continued drinking. However, the sourness of the lemon is diluted enough by the water not to create an overwhelming lip-puckering sensation of sourness.

Just don't add sugar, of course. Because if you do, you run into the enormous problems seen in the previous chapters:

The Sweet Tooth, Parts 1, 2 and 3

Children's food demands: do you have to give in?

**How much?**

A good rule of thumb for water consumption is to take your weight in pounds and divide by 2. Drink that many ounces per day. For example, a 140 lb. person needs 70 ounces of water everyday. Be sure to carry it with you when you're out and about, so you don't get home so dehydrated at night that you then have to make up for lost time and then go to bed with a rapidly filling bladder. Start drinking water first thing in the morning before breakfast.

# Chapter 24
# Codex Alimentarius: are we still allowed to choose our own food?

In 1994, after enormous consumer pressure on Congress, the Dietary Supplement and Health Education Act (DSHEA) was passed. Since then, the U.S. public has enjoyed free access to a gamut of safe, legal and affordable vitamins, minerals, amino acids, Omega-3 oils and numerous other supplements.

Now, the World Trade Organization (WTO) and its arm the Codex Alimentarius Commission, with heavy pressure from a number of European countries as well as the pharmaceutical industry, seek to limit that access in the markets of all WTO member countries. The Codex has been assigned the rather tyrannical task of establishing international guidelines for foods, supposedly to protect consumers and facilitate trade among WTO member nations.

The proposed regulations would strongly limit the potency of supplements. For example, Vitamin C over 200 mg would be available by prescription only. Furthermore, the World Health Organization (WHO) is requiring technical dossiers or "monographs" of each supplement sold. Very few such documents are being produced though because of the great expense of doing so. Such a legal maneuver is most perilous for the generally small nutraceutical companies, but of course, could be accomplished within the budgets of the global pharmaceutical giants.

Part of the rationale offered for tight worldwide regulation of supplements is that the WHO and many of the world's largest economies continue to insist on trade harmonization laws. As global trade increases, this becomes ever more the case. Robert Verkerk, PhD of the Alliance for Natural Health asks, "But which harmonization standards should be applied? Those of countries with a long-held and very restricted view on dietary supplements (e.g. Germany, France, Denmark) or which have traditionally been more liberal, such as the USA, South Africa, UK and the Netherlands?"[1]

The other rationale for imposing such restrictions is safety. Although nutritional supplements have an extraordinarily good safety record, having been shown to be even safer than foods, the safety of supplements is ever more frequently called into question. The bogus Vitamin E criticism[2] of 2005 made top of the news in

---

[1] Robert Verkerk BSc MSc DIC PhD, Executive Director, Alliance for Natural Health, "Leading US doctors endorse Alliance for Natural Health."

[2] Miller ER; Pastor-Barriuso, Dalal D, Riemersma RA, Appel LA, Guallar E. Meta-analysis: High-dosage Vitamin E supplementation may increase all-cause mortality. *Annals of Internal Medicine*, 2005; 142(1), in press. (electronic version: www.annals.org/cgi/content/full/0000605-200501040-00110v1). See rebuttal by the Alliance for Natural

the U.S. for a few days, yet 55,000 were killed by Merck's drug Vioxx, and neither Merck nor their legal arm, the U.S. Food and Drug Administration (FDA) have gotten more than a slap on the wrist. Dr. Wallace Heath remarks "106,000 hospitalized patients per year (290 per day!) die from adverse drug reactions, and two million more need more hospitalization for recovery. These were FDA approved drugs, properly administered by competent professionals in hospitals! This is the fourth highest cause of death in the U.S., accounting for 7% of all hospitalized patients. This is equivalent to a 9-11 attack every ten days. There are ***no*** fatalities from supplements, except for when Ephedra was combined with toxic stimulants by a handful of individuals, or the news would be on every front page. There is no need for more FDA control of supplements than is already in place, which is substantial. Instead of drastically restricting supplements, why doesn't the FDA better control and restrict the extremely dangerous pharmaceutical drugs which are now killing the hospitalized and non-hospitalized at the rate of a major airline crash per day?" Combining hospital deaths from drugs with non-hospital deaths from pharmaceutical drugs results in the leading cause of death in the U.S..

**Codex Alimentarius Update and H.R. 3156**

Due to mass somnolence, complacency and inertia, more of our rights have in 2006 been removed from us. The Codex Alimentarius Commission met in Rome to ratify their vitamin and mineral supplement standards as *the* international standard. This means that WTO, which its member nations have given the authority to enforce global compliance with all Codex standards, can impose trade sanctions on non-compliant nations. Such vaguely large and powerful entities can reach all the way into your local health food store and affect what was previously a harmless

---

Healthat: www.alliance-natural-health.org/index.cfm?action=news&ID=112

arrangement of free will among you, the health food store proprietor and the nutritional supplement manufacturer.

Some of the problems with Codex, aside from the travesty of taking away individuals' right to nourish themselves as they see fit and replacing the sovereign individual with a bureaucrat's views on nutrition is the following:[44]

Codex will define the maximum allowable doses of any permitted nutrients, whatever that turns out to be, while the minimum allowable dosages are 15% of the amount naturally occurring in foods. No dosage exceeding the permitted upper limit may be used, with or without a prescription. Higher doses of permitted nutrients and any dose of a nutrient not specifically permitted would be illegal under any circumstances.

Now that Codex is the official international standard for dietary supplements, it is only a matter of time before the U.S. Congress, faced with a choice of actually representing the American people, or taking the usual low road of bowing to their generous pharmaceutical lobbyist benefactors, will probably try to dismantle DSHEA and replace it with Codex standards.

Here is what the U.S Constitution has to say about such affronts to our liberty:

U.S. Constitution, Article VI: "This Constitution, and the Laws of the United States which shall be made in Pursuance thereof; and all Treaties made, or which shall be made, under the Authority of the United States, shall be the supreme Law of the Land; and the Judges in every State shall be bound thereby, any Thing in the

[44] Ostrolenk, Michael. Codex Alimentarius, Nutritional Supplements and Consumer Freedom. AAPS News. American Association of Physicians and Surgeons. Washington DC. August 2005. p S1

Constitution or Laws of any State to the Contrary notwithstanding."

Now if the American people would simply inform our elected representatives that they will just have to suffer WTO trade sanctions for being so ignorant and corrupt as to allow Codex misdeeds in the first place, and that we adamantly uphold our rights to nourish ourselves as we see fit, then we just may be able to beat this thing.

**H.R. 3156**

Losing no time at all in attacking nutritional supplements, Representatives Davis, Dingell and Waxman have introduced H.R. 3156, which they called the "Dietary Supplement Access and Awareness Act." This act defines an "adverse experience regarding a dietary supplement" to mean "any adverse event associated with the use of such supplement in humans, whether or not such event is considered to be related to the supplement . . ." (H.R. 3156, Sec. 416, (c) 4 (A).

Among sane people, cause and effect might be reasonably determined. However, such reckless wording in this political environment would allow anything from hurricane damage to a hot, spilled McDonald's coffee to be blamed on whatever dietary supplement may have been recently ingested. A pregnant woman could take a nutritional supplement the day before delivering, and then if there are birth defects or other abnormalities, it could be blamed on the supplement. For this reason alone, we have the sad situation in this country of some naturopathic physicians refusing to treat pregnant women at all, because the potential liability is too great, and natural therapies are too easily blamed by the drug-besotted FDA.

Supplements are particularly vulnerable because the FDA has most of its funding from the pharmaceutical industry, along with a revolving door between their respective human resources departments, together with some of the strongest enforcement powers in the government: such as search and seizure. This particularly bad combination has led to FDA removal of a whole class of nutritional supplements: Ephedra and all supplements containing it were banned after some one dozen individuals combined ephedra with alcohol and/or recreational drugs, which resulted in side effects.

**Codex Pharmaceuticus?**

Instead of regulating harmless vitamins, minerals and other substances, it would seem more prudent to issue guidelines limiting the use of pharmaceuticals, which are still the leading cause of death in the United States, killing more people every day than heart disease and cancer

Major problems with pharmaceuticals include:

1. Toxic side effects, which lead to further prescription of other medications, with further toxic side effects, spiraling downward to severe disease and death. Many people never again achieve their natural homeostasis or mental-emotional health after even a few doses of certain pharmaceuticals. Xanax is a popular drug that after a few doses leaves people even years later with the sensation of "never being the same again."

2. The deadly combination of ubiquitous pharmaceuticals and ubiquitous cars. Because of drugged-out drivers, other drivers, passengers and pedestrians are unsafe.

3. Massive recreational abuse of prescription pharmaceuticals. Oxycontin parties were all the rage a decade ago. Now teens are engaging in "pharming parties" where one teen trades Ritalin for another's Percodan, or Vicodin or Xanax. The problem is attracting the attention of the medical profession. Dr. Francis Hayden, Director of the Adolescent Mental Health Center at Mount Sinai Hospital in New York says, "When adults and medical professionals treat medications casually, we need not be surprised that adolescents are treating them casually."[45] The good news is that use of illegal substances such as speed and pot have declined over the past decade, in large part due to the disincentive of jail time. Bad news is that heroin use is now more widespread, and the recreational drugs of choice include prescription pharmaceuticals, which have created their own class of drug abusers, mostly among partying teens. Columbia University's National Center on Addiction and Substance Abuse (CASA) has stated that 2.3 million kids ages 12 to 17 took legal medications illegally in 2003, the latest year for which the figures are tallied. That's three times the number in 1992, or about 1 of every 10 teens.[46]

Part of the problem is addiction: Such drugs as Xanax, Valium, Vicodin, Ritalin and Adderall are highly addictive. The stimulant properties of drugs like Ritalin and Adderall, prescribed for kids with hyperactivity or short attention spans, have left many of them seeking similar effects from methamphetamines once they outgrow their Ritalin prescriptions.

---

[45] Banta, Carolyn. Trading for a High. Newsweek. August 1, 2005. p. 35.
[46] Banta. Ibid.

Another problem is that when such drugs are used recreationally, rather than as prescribed, a visit to the emergency room is all the more likely.

Given the reckless use of pharmaceuticals in our society, perhaps guidelines should be issued for their use, rather than for such harmless items as nutritional supplements.

The Food and Drug Administration, which is responsible for such regulation, ignores those duties because of their close ties with the pharmaceutical industry. Those ties were made much closer in 1992 when Congress passed a law with no debate that increased the FDA's dependence on large drug companies for its funding.[47] The FDA is simply a trade association for the pharmaceutical industry with the added power of having the force of the federal government behind it. Then a majority of FDA officials go on to very high-paying jobs with the pharmaceutical giants after a stint at the FDA. So much drug money and incentives for that money has flowed through the FDA that to assume the FDA is qualified to impartially judge drugs, foods, supplements or anything else is ludicrous.

Therefore, an initiative for Codex Pharmaceuticus is not likely to come from the powers that be any time soon, but wouldn't it make an appropriate response to the unethical and intolerable Codex Alimentarius?

---

[47] Trudeau, Kevin. *Natural cures "they" don't want you to know about.* Alliance Publishing Group. 2004.

# Chapter 25
# Traveling with Good Food

Even if you have an excellent fresh diet of whole organic food at home, that can all fall apart while traveling. Relying on restaurants and markets away from home is often a disappointing experience. The problem is worse as we move from the large cities out toward the suburbs and hits bottom in the rural areas.

In large cities and suburbs, when perusing the yellow pages for restaurants, keep in mind that large health food stores often have good cafés inside, although with hours limited to the store's hours or shorter. College towns and the commercial streets near universities will often have some of the healthiest eateries in proximity to some of the most decadent. Also consider ethnic neighborhoods and restaurants for gastric relief from burger-and-fries purgatory.

**Most challenging: traveling in rural areas**

With some of the richest topsoil in the world, America's heartland should be replete with markets, roadside stands and restaurants overflowing with abundant choices of fresh harvest from neighboring farmland. Instead we see some of the most dismal offerings of food in the heartland. Because of the monoculture fields and far flung distribution patterns, your only choices at Homer's Truckstop may be little more than defrosted beef or pork, canned corn or peas, assembly-line fries and of course desserts. Rural markets are not much better.

Your best bet for decent food in rural areas is the increasingly rare roadside produce stand or farmers' market. Also, if you happen to travel to areas where there is community-supported agriculture, these farms are a welcome relief to monoculture. Although they are committed to first filling orders for their regular local subscribers, their excess harvest often ends up in local markets or at their own produce stands. http://www.localharvest.org is a web resource for community supported farms, as well as farmers' markets, healthy restaurants and food co-ops throughout the U.S.

Traveling by car rather than by plane makes eating what you want a bit easier, because you can more easily carry a cooler in the trunk. One thing you can count on at rural stores and truck stops is plenty of ice. If you have small children, you will also need small containers, utensils and a paring knife, so you can cut whatever fresh fruits and vegetables are available into chunks for them, and store the containers in the cooler. For car trips, pack leftovers from home that will keep for a few days, and that you would not mind eating cold if necessary.

Many people make the mistake of drinking water from plastic bottles, and leaving them on hot sunny car seats. The danger in this is that the heat drives the plasticizers right into the water, where they act as xenoestrogens – like female hormones, only much worse and much more carcinogenic. These are really, really bad for men and women and especially children. Instead, the next time you're in a health food store, buy any beverage in glass bottles of a convenient size. Ice tea often comes in glass. Then save the bottles, at least one for each family member, to reuse indefinitely. Glass bottles if kept clean can be left on a hot car seat or any other relatively benign place with no harm to the water, because of the inert chemical nature of glass.

A soft-sided cooler works better when traveling by plane so that it can fit in carry-on spaces. A regular cooler is harder to carry on a plane because most coolers won't fit under the seats or in overhead bins. But if you want to have it for the road later, wrap the cooler with packaging tape, and check it. For the flight, pack the soft-sided cooler or a sturdy bag as a carry-on with enough home-made food and utensils for the day that you don't have to rely on abysmal airline offerings. Nutrient-dense foods like nuts pack small. Apples, cheese, carrots, cucumbers and celery stalks filled with nut butter or goat cheese are examples of other easy finger food that all balance each other nutritionally. All of it gets irradiated of course in the airport, which has been in my experience unavoidable and non-negotiable since 9/11.

Staying at a hotel with kitchenette facilities frees you from complete dependence on restaurants, which is advantageous because of the greater choices in supermarket food than restaurant menu options. This is easiest if you stay in one place for most of your trip. However, if you are traveling from one town to another every day or two, use the kitchen facilities to replenish your store of leftovers in stackable containers in your cooler, leaning especially toward fast, non-complicated recipes that don't need a lot of esoteric spices or other possibly expensive ingredients, and that you would not mind having cold for lunch if necessary. The more you change hotels the harder this becomes as your refrigeration space is limited to that of your cooler.

Perhaps most importantly, when traveling don't suffer quietly with the pathetic food offerings of your unenlightened hosts. Speak up to the servers at the restaurants or the clerks in the supermarkets: Aren't there any fresh vegetables available? Why don't they carry grass-fed beef? Alaskan wild salmon? Free-range organic chicken? It should make them wonder why they settle for second-rate food for themselves. There is a certain Tex-Mex restaurant chain that shall remain nameless, where I happened to visit once with a party of about twelve several years ago. I asked the server if the guacamole was made fresh, to which she answered, "It's canned." I'm afraid I did not hide my horror very well when I repeated "It's *canned*???" which startled the whole table. (Imagine canning the quickly perishable avocado.) Anyway, that particular chain now offers fresher and much better tasting guacamole. I certainly don't flatter myself that I alone changed a policy of a national restaurant chain; as an anonymous, ordinary-looking person, I'm sure I was a little drop in a big bucket. But enough other customers must have commented similarly. Our *combined* voices, each demanding better-quality food of our cardboard-slinging restaurants and supermarkets can conceivably attain such **impact** as the very broad-based "slow food" movement is achieving in Europe. Especially when traveling, just remember that old rule of the road: it's the squeaky wheel that gets the grease. That is to say, the healthy zeal gets roast geese.

# Chapter 26
# What's so great about Community Supported Agriculture?

CSA is a rapidly growing movement of family farms that work directly with consumers. Local consumers take a "share" or subscription in their nearby farm's harvest of just-picked produce (or dairy, eggs, chicken, beef, etc.). In exchange for an annual fee, subscribers reap the fresh harvest every week straight off the farm. In fact, CSA farms grow specifically for their community. The farms involved are family farms on small acreages. Farm products are often organic, as requested by the consumers, and therefore much easier on the environment.

The environmental benefits are many. In the United States, small farmers devote 17% of their area to woodlands, compared to only 5% on large farms. Small farms maintain nearly twice as much of their land in "soil improving uses," including cover crops and green manures.

But there are social and economic benefits as well: In farming communities dominated by large corporate farms, nearby towns are dying off. The empty ghost towns of our prairie states and other farming regions are what agribusiness has left of once thriving towns with busy main streets. Where family farms predominate, on the other hand, there are more local businesses, schools, parks, churches, clubs, and newspapers, as well as better services, higher employment, and more civic participation. Furthermore, the smallest U.S. farms, those of 27 acres or less, have more than ten times greater dollar output per acre than larger farms, thereby requiring less acreage on which to feed the same number of people.

But the most wonderful thing about community-supported agriculture is the appreciation it gives us of the earth-source of our food. Rather than boxing and packaging every product and even the consumer behind a wall of ignorance, CSA brings the beauty, immediacy and intimacy of our earth into all of the food that we receive from the farms. The fresh, delicious taste and fragrance of the recently harvested produce is beyond comparison with the supermarket inventories that sit for several days in their massive piles waiting for purchase. Compare just harvested produce with canned soup, for example in which the vegetables are over two years old on average.

For a CSA farm in your area, see the directory at www.localharvest.org or www.csacenter.org.

# Part III
# Finding a doctor who knows these things, and who understands health as much as disease

# Chapter 27
# Naturopathic physicians

Naturopathy is essentially an eclectic system of medicine using the most natural and least invasive methods of treating disease. Yet it is not so much a collection of treatment strategies as it is a philosophy of treating. Naturopathic physician Kenneth Proefrock, NMD, says: "What defines naturopathic physicians is not so much the substances they use, but how they use them. Naturopathic doctors will even at times prescribe pharmaceuticals if it will help restore some sense of balance so that the patient can then go on to achieve a higher level of health."

The biggest difference with conventional "allopathic" medicine is this approach to the patient. *Allo* (opposite) *pathy* (disease) fights symptoms with substances that are opposite in function and suppress those symptoms. Naturopathic physicians, in contrast, are far more interested in how a person got to feel ill in the first place, and identifying that first cause of disease and correcting that cause, so that the resulting symptoms are then eliminated. Sometimes, symptom suppression is necessary regardless of the form of medicine, but naturopaths see that as only a means to an end. For example, if a person is in so much pain that they can't function or enjoy life, then pain relief would be appropriate until the underlying cause of the pain is eliminated by other means.

The six defining principles of naturopathic medicine further illustrate this philosophy and approach:

1. First do no harm
2. Nature has the power to heal
3. Treat the whole person
4. Treat the cause
5. Prevent disease
6. Doctor as teacher

"First do no harm" was Hippocrates' instruction to physicians and may be thought of as an application of The Golden Rule. Whatever intervention a doctor can make in a patient's health and life, the only acceptable action is one that will do no further damage to the patient's health. It doesn't get much more sensible than this rule first learned as toddlers: "Don't hurt anybody."

Second, naturopathic doctors rely on the healing power of nature to help restore patients to complete health. The really excellent naturopath is one who knows how to "work the modalities": that is to be able to draw from the vast materia medica of natural materials as appropriate for specific patients and to be able to apply them to the great variety and complication of illnesses that are common today, and better yet, to offer the patient a choice among multiple effective treatments.

Another principle is to treat the whole person. Naturopaths know better than to give you a medication that will calm your arthritis but leave you blind, or that will clear up the skin while skewing your hormones out of balance. Naturopaths are trained to consider the whole patient, not just the one part of the body with obvious symptoms. The job of the naturopathic doctor is to make sure that what you get is helpful and completely benign for all of you.

The fourth principle is to treat the cause. For example, you may have chronic inflammation, which has caused joint stiffness and imbalanced immune function. The naturopath goes to the cause of the problem and treats the inflammation and its cause, because when you remove the cause, the joints move more easily and the immune system improves. So that way you resolve all three problems instead of just one.

To prevent disease is another naturopathic principle. The improved lifestyle of naturopathic patients is what enables the body to regain homeostasis and to better deflect the constant stresses and toxic conditions that a heavily trafficked industrial society imposes. Our study and practice of environmental medicine teaches the importance of removing toxins from the patient's body and home. Likewise, naturopathic doctors help their patients find satisfactory ways to include healthy foods in the diet and whole food alternatives to harmful processed foods, so that preventing disease becomes an easy routine as well as a pleasant experience.

Perhaps the last principle is most important of all: it is even more important for a doctor to be a teacher than a healer. In accordance with the idea that if you give someone a fish he may eat that day, but if you teach him to fish he may eat for a lifetime, *the doctor must teach how to heal*, and how to live comfortably long-term with good quality food, sound sleep, stress reduction measures and a fun, feasible exercise program. Ultimately, the most successful patients learn to take responsibility for their own health, with the doctor acting as a resource and tutor toward that goal.

Naturopathic physicians are naturopathic doctors (ND), or naturopathic medical doctors (NMD). After graduation from a four-year college or university, naturopaths are trained in four-year medical colleges just as other physicians are. The difference is that in naturopathic medical school, in addition to learning such basic medical sciences as anatomy, physiology, biochemistry, microbiology, pathology, pharmacology, immunology, histology, neuroanatomy and genetics, naturopathic students also attend full courses in specific clinical sciences over the next two years: obstetrics, pediatrics, gynecology, urology, geriatrics, neurology, eyes-ears-nose-throat, pulmonology, cardiology, gastroenterology, endocrinology, dermatology, rheumatology and oncology. Naturopathic students take courses in standard medical procedures: physical diagnosis, laboratory diagnosis, radiology and clinical procedures (multiple courses of each) as well as emergency medicine and minor surgery. Of course, naturopaths also learn the naturopathic therapies. These include: clinical nutrition (that is, nutrition as both a healing therapy and applied biochemistry), botanical medicine (nutritive and therapeutic plants), homeopathy, Oriental Medicine such as acupuncture and herbs, as well as environmental medicine, physical medicine and hydrotherapy. Naturopaths are trained both in the classroom and in a variety of clinical settings.

Throughout the naturopathic medical curriculum, naturopaths are required to take board exams to ensure that both the training and skills come up to the standards required across North America for the naturopathic profession. Just as for medical doctors and osteopathic physicians, naturopathic physicians are required to take Continuing Education courses periodically in order to stay at peak competence.

Just be sure that you ask for a licensed ND (Naturopathic Doctor) or NMD (Naturopathic Medical Doctor), because licensed naturopaths are the ones who are both classroom and clinically trained to practice medicine. There are some health care practitioners who call themselves "naturopaths" or "traditional naturopaths" but who have never enrolled in a medical school. They may have purchased their diploma online and may have never treated anyone before you. Such people may have good intentions and want to help their fellow humans, but are at a serious loss regarding the necessary knowledge and experience to be trusted with your health. Licensed naturopathic physicians on the other hand have graduated from a four-year, on-site medical school, and have worked with several hundred patients at minimum before graduating. A naturopathic doctor's license to practice medicine is issued by one of the states listed in the next chapter, although naturopathic physicians may be found in all fifty states and abroad.

For the most part, naturopathic medicine is still not covered by most medical insurance. However, as many people have happily discovered, the out-of-pocket costs to a naturopath's patients are often much less than the out-of-pocket costs (that is deductibles and uncovered services and products) for fully insured people who go to conventional physicians and who need pharmaceuticals and/or hospital care. That is, a naturopath's tools, which are basically materials found in nature, often plant materials, are so much less expensive than patented prescription drugs that many people end up paying less even without insurance. These savings are magnified as time goes on, considering the much greater relative improvement in overall health of the naturopathic patient over the average person.

# Chapter 28
# How to choose a naturopathic physician

With only about 3,000 naturopathic physicians in the U.S., it may be hard to find one at all, let alone to be picky. Part of the difficulty is the name: In Arizona and California, they are Naturopathic Medical Doctors (NMDs) or Naturopathic Doctors (NDs). In the twelve other states[48] where naturopathic physicians are licensed, they are Naturopathic Doctors (NDs). In the

[48] Naturopathic physicians are licensed in the following states:

Alaska
Arizona
California
Connecticut
Hawaii
Idaho
Kansas
Maine
Maryland
Minnesota
Montana
New Hampshire
North Dakota
Oregon
Utah
Vermont
Washington (state)
Washington D.C.

unlicensed states, you may think you have found a naturopathic physician, but because there is no license and no regulation, you may have simply encountered a correspondence school customer, who bought a diploma saying "ND", but has never done the necessary academic and clinical work to train as a physician. In other words, the mail-order NDs may have never set foot inside a medical school. In the interest of your own health, it is best to not entrust it to such a person any more than you would entrust your health to a manicurist or a roofer. For whatever good intentions such individuals may have, they simply don't have the necessary training. Worse, their lack of training and lack of medical education from time to time produce fatal outcomes in patients. Then what the media report to the public is that a naturopath allegedly killed someone. The mail order schools usurping of our name and our diploma "Naturopathic Doctor" gives the real naturopaths a bad name and deceives and endangers the public. For that reason, licensing efforts for naturopathic medicine are underway in most states, and state legislatures are waking up to the problem. In order to avoid such an encounter yourself, make sure your ND graduated from one of the six accredited North American naturopathic medical schools in the following list:

Bastyr University (U.S.) (campuses in WA and CA)
Boucher Institute of Naturopathic Medicine (candidate for accreditation, Canada)
Canadian College of Naturopathic Medicine (Canada)
National College of Natural Medicine (U.S.)
National University of Health Sciences (U.S.)
Southwest College of Naturopathic Medicine (U.S.)
University of Bridgeport College of Naturopathic Medicine (candidate for accreditation, U.S.)

These are the only seven naturopathic medical schools accredited by the Council on Naturopathic Medical Education (CNME). A copy of the doctor's diploma from one of these six schools should be hanging in his or her office. Before making the appointment, find out what school the ND graduated from, and don't let anybody tell you about other naturopathic schools. There are no other accredited schools in the U.S. and Canada, and no other on-site naturopathic medical curricula with clinical training programs apart from these seven. Period. Naturopathic Doctors from these seven medical schools complete more hours of in-class and laboratory medical training than any other type of physician, including MDs and DOs, and our total hours of academic plus clinical training are comparable to such medical schools as Yale School of Medicine and the osteopathic schools. This data is also kept by the U.S. Department of Education.

Yet another problem once you have found an accredited ND is that there are some who are afraid to practice naturopathic medicine, and feel as if they need to conform to their conventional medical colleagues by practicing conventional medicine. Here are two questions to weed out such individuals:

1) "Do you follow the therapeutic order for naturopathic medicine?" The therapeutic order emphasizes the importance of using natural treatments first, before resorting to conventional medical treatments, except in the case of most emergencies. If the ND doesn't know how to answer this question, you should perhaps raise one eyebrow.
2) "Do you consider yourself a vitalist? How do you use vitalism in your practice?" A vitalist is one who relies on such lifestyle changes as nutrition, sleep, exercise, elimination, detoxification, water therapy, physical manipulation and stress management as important treatment tools for every patient, and the only treatment tools for some patients. Once these matters are addressed, such natural treatments as botanical medicines, acupuncture or homeopathy are employed. Only in certain

medical conditions are pharmaceuticals or surgery necessary. If this question seems to perplex or tongue-tie the ND, or if you sense that you are not getting an honest, straightforward response, you should probably raise the other eyebrow too, and maybe even find a more helpful naturopathic physician in the future. Naturopathic physicians in your area may be found from an internet search or at www.naturopathic.org.

# Chapter 29
# Homeopaths and homeopathic physicians

The first part of this series discussed naturopathy, an eclectic system of medicine that includes homeopathy, botanical medicine, nutrition, and several other fields of medicine with a principle of using the most appropriate substances or procedures that an individual patient with an individual symptom picture and constitution may need most in order to achieve lasting improved health.

Dr. Samuel Hahnemann, the founder of homeopathy, received his medical degree from the University of Erlangen in Bavaria in 1799, emerging into an era when bloodletting and leeches were the norm for medical treatments. In contrast, Hahnemann maintained such radical ideas as keeping one's precious blood, sensible diet, regular exercise and sufficient sleep, as well as humane treatment for the mentally ill, who were at the time generally confined to cellars and physically abused. He was so far ahead of his time that he was met with opposition and disdain from other physicians, a pattern that continued throughout his life.

Hahnemann's first patient for homeopathic experimentation was himself. He noticed that when he sampled the malaria medication cinchona he acquired symptoms very similar to malaria. Hahnemann recorded his observations as follows: "Cinchona bark, which is used as a remedy for the intermittent fever [malaria] acts because it can produce symptoms similar to those of intermittent fever in healthy people." Here Hahnemann has described a central principle of homeopathy, the Law of Similars. It says that the substance that is most curative for a disease condition is the one that would produce symptoms most similar to that disease in a healthy person.

The opposite nature of conventional medicine and homeopathy is reflected in their names. "Homeopathy" is from the Greek, meaning similar suffering, or similar disease state. "Allopathy" or conventional Western medicine is also from the Greek, meaning opposite suffering. Whereas allopathic medicine gives opposites to produce relief of symptoms, homeopathy gives a similar substance. Let's look at the example of insomnia: an allopath (a M.D. usually) might offer a sleeping pill for insomnia. This would produce a sedative or sleepy effect to overwhelm the body and mind's tendency to wakefulness. In this case, the sedative is somewhat stronger than the wakeful impulse of the patient, and for the time being at least, sleep is achieved.

In contrast, a homeopath might use coffee as a remedy for insomnia. Although coffee is everywhere considered to be a stimulant, for homeopaths it is actually sedative in its effect, when it is homeopathically diluted, not full-strength coffee (which is certainly stimulating). How can coffee possibly relieve insomnia? Here is how homeopathic remedies work: homeostasis is the perfect, happy condition of our bodies. Homeostasis involves just the right temperature, the right sweating, the right appetite and thirst, the right energy-rest cycles, the right hormone balance, and so many other mechanisms for our optimal functioning. Our bodies are so constantly striving to achieve, sometimes even desperate to achieve, homeostasis that we are constantly in pursuit of this wonderful and normal condition. Sometimes, however, one or more homeostatic parameters, say the sleep-wake cycle, is out of whack. Often it needs just a bit of a stimulus to prime our homeostatic mechanisms to come back to optimal levels. Homeopathic coffee, for some insomnia patients, can provide just this push, or irritant, or little alarm prompting to bring the system back to homeostasis (i.e., to alleviate the insomnia.) The cure thus achieved lasts longer and more thoroughly than allopathic treatment, because the homeopathic stimulus caused the body itself to create the cure, rather than simply to temporarily suppress the symptoms. Thus, for children who are too active late in the evening, a dose of homeopathic coffee often helps them get right to sleep. Because homeopathic doses are so dilute, there is little or no primary pharmacological effect (in this case, stimulant), and only the rebound or secondary effect remains (in this case, sedative) after the patient's hypothalamus has sensed stimulation and corrects it back to homeostasis.

Homeopathy may be the most misunderstood of all systems of medicine. The most confusing and controversial aspect of homeopathy is the Law of the Minimum Dose. According to this thinking, the more diluted the homeopathic preparation, the more powerfully it works. We know that with pharmaceutical drugs, the more one takes, generally the more powerful the effect up to a certain maximum. How then could it be the opposite in homeopathy? How can you dilute a substance till it's pretty much all gone, and then claim that it works? The answer to this question is still quite up in the air. Mostly homeopaths and satisfied homeopathic patients tend to respond, "well, it just works. You just have to see it for yourself." But this empirical answer has never satisfied scientists or physicians trained in the scientific model or other scientifically minded or skeptically thinking people.

Other hypotheses do exist however. Current thinking is that when one dilutes in the specific homeopathic method of dilution, which involves successive dilution with pure distilled water, as well as succussion, or shaking, the water molecules create patterns, like snowflakes, unique and precise, around each molecule of solute. In other words, a homeopathic dilution of sulfur and a homeopathic preparation of oyster shell look pretty much the same to the casual observer: just water. But that water is very different, in that one has the "imprint" of the sulfur, and the other resembles, in its properties and molecular mega-structures or "clathrates," the "imprint" of the oyster shell. Each is just as precise and repetitive in its own way as the intricate six-sided symmetry of a snowflake, yet each is as distinct as one snowflake is from another. And this has been show in laboratory experiments, verified by infrared imaging and nuclear magnetic resonance. Yet another snowflake-like imprint could be made of a homeopathic dilution of phosphorus or squid ink or sunflower or platinum. Each homeopathic solute or "mother tincture" (the starting substance) is used by homeopathic pharmacists to create the unique homeopathically "imprinted" water, which is then sprayed onto the neutral homeopathic pillules of powdered lactose that are taken by the patient. This enables the specific imprint of the mother tincture to be maintained and transferred in such a vehicle that it can arrive to the patient's bloodstream intact.

**As always, treat the whole person**

Naturopaths who practice homeopathy take some of the most thoroughly detailed patient histories of any type of health care practitioner. Whereas allopathic doctors may certainly prescribe certain drugs for certain conditions, i.e., sleeping pills for insomnia, in homeopathy your doctor must know what is happening with all of you. Homeopathic prescription is based on the totality of symptoms, rather than a single symptom. For example, the person who has trouble falling asleep at night would most likely require a different homeopathic remedy than the one who falls asleep easily but then ends up wide awake and restless in the middle of the night. Even the last category could be broken down into one who wakes with bad dreams or wakes with diarrhea or wakes feeling chilly or wakes sweating or wakes with a headache. Each of these point to different homeopathic remedies, which are generally not interchangeable among different types of insomniacs.

For this reason, it is not helpful for one to self-prescribe and choose one's own homeopathic remedy at the local health food store. You are much more likely to get the one suitable remedy, the one that best fits your present state of health vs. illness, if you let your naturopathic doctor or homeopath take your thorough case history and prescribe accordingly. Follow-up is also very important in homeopathy, because symptom pictures often change remarkably after initial intake. Work with your naturopath patiently. Healing occurs in stages (or in layers, as homeopaths like to say). The homeopathic remedy that works well for you now may well give rise to another one before you feel completely cured.

# Chapter 30
# Osteopathic physicians, Doctors of Osteopathy (D.O.)

The first part of this series discussed naturopathy, an eclectic system of medicine that includes homeopathy, botanical medicine, nutrition, and several other fields of medicine with a principle of using the most appropriate substances or procedures that an individual patient with an individual symptom picture and constitution may need most in order to achieve lasting improved health.

The second part discussed homeopathy, a system of medicine involving highly dilute amounts of substances chosen for the resemblance to the patient's disease state, according to the Law of Similars. Although homeopathy sounds so dilute as to be placebo to the uninitiated, it has been practiced with great healing effect in many countries for about 200 years.

This chapter addresses osteopathy, originally a philosophy and practice of physical medicine, which has grown more toward conventional medicine in its development as a profession. Whereas allopathic medical schools award their graduates the degree of medical doctor (M.D.), osteopathic medical schools award the Doctor of Osteopathy (D.O.). The training of these two types of physician is very similar in almost every respect: a foundation in the basic medical sciences, clinical training in all of the basic specialties of medicine, then as newly minted doctors, residencies of 3, 4 or more years in the chosen specialty. Both MDs and DOs are trained in allopathic medicine: drug treatments primarily, as well as surgery. However, osteopathic education offers its students something in addition to standard allopathic medicine. That is a system of treating the musculoskeletal system by a hands-on manipulation that is remarkable for both its gentleness and successful effect.

Most DO's today do not practice osteopathic manipulation, unfortunately, and one is about as likely to find a naturopathic physician or chiropractor who knows how to use this system. If you look for a physician who practices this manipulation, you will almost certainly have to ask the doctor's front desk staff, because it is not so widely known. Nevertheless, osteopathic manipulation is now again a required part of the osteopathic curriculum, after having been ignored for several decades, as the influence of allopathic medicine almost completely eclipsed interest in all branches of natural medicine throughout much of the last century.

Traditional osteopathic philosophy recognizes the neuro-musculoskeletal system as crucially important to the full expression and effortless use of the body and mind, and that this system is intricately connected with all other body systems and mirrors both health and disease. When the muscles and bones are not functioning well, the mind cannot be happy either.

Andrew Taylor Still, founder of osteopathy, began reflecting on the musculoskeletal system as a young boy in the 1830's, during which time he suffered from severe headaches. In order to relieve them, he learned to rest the back of his head on a rope swing that his father had hung in the yard. Still would take a nap in that position and wake up with no headache. We now know that he was applying a direct tissue technique to stretch the muscles originating at the occiput or base of the head. As these muscles stretched, the tension on them and thus the cranial bones eased sufficiently to stop pain signals in the associated nerves.

Still's intuitive understanding of his headache treatment mechanism began his lifelong interest in achievement of physical wellbeing by means of precisely applied physical manipulation. Still's ideas were rejected by the standard medical establishment, and he thus chose to establish a parallel but quite different medical educational system that he called osteopathy. In 1892, Still started the first osteopathic medical school in Kirksville, Missouri.

Today, a variety of direct tissue techniques, such as the one described above are used on the torso and extremities in order to stretch out muscles in spasm.

However, the real genius of osteopathy lies in the indirect tissue techniques, muscle energy and counterstrain. The practice of these is counterintuitive, because they take the patient's contracted or sore muscle to a position that is even shorter and as relaxed as possible. The position is the opposite of a stretched position. Conventional thinking assumes that a contracted muscle should be stretched (or dosed with a muscle relaxing drug). Traditional osteopathic thinking is the opposite: if a sore muscle is held in its most relaxed and easy position, for varying lengths of time, depending on the technique, it will tend to release the spasm of fibers that is causing shortness or tightness in that muscle. These techniques are practiced quietly, without "bone cracking," or other fanfare, but they leave the patient surprised and impressed by their curative effect and usually relieved of pain.

The difference between the muscle energy and counterstrain techniques is that counterstrain simply holds the patient in a position where the body is somewhat folded around the sore muscle for a certain period of time in order to encourage the release of muscle spasm, whereas muscle energy uses the patient's exertion opposing the physician's exertion in a way that deliberately shortens the muscle with periodic rests in between such exercises. Both these techniques may be thought of as tricking a shortened, painful muscle into allowing the release of spasm and hence decreasing pressure on the local nerves and thus allowing relief of pain as well as greater range of motion. The osteopathic physician's extensive training in anatomy and visualization of muscle fiber direction and length guide the choice of technique and the exact placement and direction of muscle shortening and lengthening.

Even for very tightly contracted muscles the use of these techniques are relatively painless compared to daily activities using such a strained muscle.

In order to find an osteopathic physician that practices osteopathic manipulation, we recommend consulting this directory of osteopaths:

http://www.holisticmed.com/www/osteopract.html.

You may also find that your local naturopathic physician or chiropractor or massage therapist may practice traditional osteopathic manipulation.

# Part IV
# What good food and other natural therapies can help you accomplish

# Chapter 31
# Youthful celebrities at 60

What do laypeople know about nutrition? Perhaps some know quite a bit as evidenced by keeping themselves healthy. On the other hand, Andrew Weil, MD, the famous alternative medicine expert, has castigated conventional medical schools for not teaching nutrition, and for churning out physicians who are ignorant of basic food-body interactions. Weil said, "The current state of nutrition education of health professionals is non-existent to substandard." As little as our doctors have helped us make good food choices over the years, we have had to learn to make our own best choices.

Having been left to our own inner wisdom for dietary choices, many people have chosen poorly, and many others have chosen well. But the anonymous and barely visible "man in the street" is difficult for researchers to observe over many decades. Whatever he has been eating for his entire life is largely forgotten, even by himself, and the course of his health and wellbeing over that time are equally unknowable. For that reason we devote this chapter to the food choices of highly visible celebrities who are more observable.

Some of the most divergent food choices are made by famous people. And fortunately, because of their broadly displayed lives, we can watch and learn the effects over time of their food choices on their bodies, their activities and their longevity. We have seen famous entertainers on the one hand who eat, drink, smoke and inject some of the most noxious substances available to them, and then burn out and expire at an untimely age.

Then there are those celebrities, notably Suzanne Somers, Goldie Hawn, Cheryl Tiegs, Christie Brinkley and others, who have maintained great health and amazingly youthful faces and bodies while choosing healthy foods and, fortunately, sharing their food choices with us.

Hawn and Somers are both in their 60s, Tiegs and Brinkley are in their 50s. All four avoid sugar and other refined carbohydrates. Goldie Hawn follows a wheat-free, sugar-free and dairy-free diet. Suzanne Somers in her Somersizing Diet Book explains why sugar, not fat is responsible for weight gain. As do so many healthy people, Somers shops the periphery of supermarkets: vegetables, fruits, dairy and meat, and that's it. Her focus is: "keeping myself healthy internally so that it manifests on the external."

Many people, on learning about the negative health effects of sugar, think, "I just can't give it up."

Here is what Suzanne Somers has to say about "can't":

"I will not start any sentence with the words, "I can't." If I do, my mind will accept it as so, and then I won't be able to accomplish my goals. Instead I will tell myself, "I can," or "I will." In this way success will come to me."

Even more remarkably, Somers was diagnosed with breast cancer in 2001. She made headlines at the time for choosing homeopathic treatment over chemotherapy, and has survived healthfully. Undoubtedly, her diet played a role, because sugar feeds cancer. In fact, glucose is the number one fuel for cancer, and Somers decided to deprive cancer of that fuel.

Certainly, the above-mentioned celebrities never attended medical school, nor studied the intricate details of biochemistry to appreciate just how health-destroying sugar is, or how necessary whole foods are. But from the available evidence of their youthfulness into the sixth and seventh decades, it's not rocket science to figure out that they've been doing something impeccably correct -- they've been treating their bodies in such a way as to enjoy every part of a long life. To me - and I am a doctor, with 4 years of medical school training, a preceptorship, an internship and over 80 published health and nutrition articles behind me - this life experience, this putting their own wellbeing on the line, and demonstrating the results over decades of public life, makes them much better teachers of nutrition than those conventional doctors who struggled or half-dozed through biochemistry in med school, while never really understanding its impact on our lives. It seems clear who the better health experts are.

However, in order to get from here to there, it is often helpful to consult with a naturopathic physician or other natural health care provider, such as Dr. Joseph Mercola, who do have extensive knowledge of nutrition. Together with such a physician, you can determine an eating plan that is right for you, and that you will find satisfying while working toward your weight and health goals. Dr. Mercola may be found in Schaumberg, IL, or on his website, www.Mercola.com, which is the largest natural health website in the U.S., with a free newsletter of practical health-related information. In order to locate a naturopathic physician near you, we recommend consulting the database of the American Association of Naturopathic Physicians, at http://www.naturopathic.org.

# Chapter 32
# Why light matters

Bone health is greatly dependent on quality light. We make Vitamin D through our skin when exposed to optimal levels of sunlight. Vitamin D is key to a proper quantity and balance of calcium and magnesium in the body, as well as a healthy balance of hormones. A growing body of research demonstrates that by increasing one's exposure to full spectrum light it is possible to optimize hormone levels in the body. Such balance is key to avoiding osteoporosis and fractures, as well as minimizing tooth decay.

Recent research has confirmed the essential role of Vitamin D in such necessary function as insulin secretion, cancer prevention, bone health and hormone formation.

Historically, osteoporosis and age-related fractures have hit hardest at those populations who stay in the dark. Contemporary

Americans and Europeans who stay indoors much of the time have much higher rates of hip and other fractures than people whose lifestyle kept them outdoors or dependent on natural light. Only a century ago, we had no light bulbs at all, and we had no fluorescent lights until 50 years ago.

A nine-month long study of first grade children in windowless classrooms found that those under full-spectrum fluorescent lights had many fewer cavities in their newly formed permanent teeth than those under standard "cool white" fluorescent bulbs. It turned out that ten times as many children under cool white bulbs had new cavities ($p<0.005$)[49]. Many fewer cavities were also found when incandescent bulbs, which are higher in red and infrared, were used instead of full-spectrum fluorescent bulbs. The authors also found that a broad spectrum of ultraviolet, red and infrared light was important for the formation of teeth as well as resistance to decay.

Animal studies have confirmed this. Hamsters placed under cool white bulbs 12 hours per day for fifteen weeks had five times more cavities and ten times greater tooth loss per cavity (a total of 50 times greater tooth loss) than those hamsters placed under fluorescent bulbs with ultraviolet added to approximate natural sunlight.

Furthermore, the development of the male sexual organs was only one fifth as great in those hamsters under cool white light as compared to those under full spectrum light. Of course, this result correlates with our knowledge that testosterone, a steroid

[49] Mayron, Ott, Amontree and Nations, "Caries reduction in school children." Applied Radiology. July/Aguust 1975. pp.56-58.

hormone, is dependent on Vitamin D for its synthesis, a Vitamin that we make from sunlight.[50]

It has also been found that the role of full-spectrum light benefits the eyes as well as when it strikes the skin. The natural light received by the eyes plays a vital role in body chemistry. The light received by the eyes influences the hypothalamus, which in turn influences the pituitary and pineal glands. The pineal gland especially is involved in our diurnal rhythms, and our lack of quality light through the retina may be the source of many sleep disorders that are increasingly common among people who are always indoors.

Much research on this subject is summarized by the German ophthalmologist Fritz Hollwich, MD[51] as well as by John Ott, Hon. D. Sci. a researcher on the properties of light.[52] The array of bodily organs and systems that depend on full-spectrum light through the eyes is astounding. When the eyes are exposed to natural sunlight or full-spectrum light, the pituitary gland, thyroid gland, adrenal glands, ovaries, testes, pancreas, liver and kidneys all function better, according to the numerous studies presented in these two books. Full-spectrum light includes a balance of wavelengths from all colors of the visible spectrum plus ultraviolet and infrared. On the other hand, cool white fluorescent bulbs, which are now used for the great majority of interior commercial lighting, have strong yellow, but are very deficient in most of the other wavelengths, with no ultraviolet or infrared.

---

[50] Sharon, Feller and Burney. "The effects of lights of different spectra on caries incidence in the golden hamster." Archives of Oral Biology. Vol 1, No. 12 1971. pp. 1427-1432.
[51] Fritz Hollwich MD. *The Influence of Ocular Light Perception on Metabolism in Man and Animal.* Springer Verlag. New York. 1979.
[52] John Ott D. Sci Hon.. *Health and Light.* Devin Adair Co. 1976.

Unfortunately, however, UV light has received a bad name, primarily because of individuals who have a history of blistering sunburns followed by skin cancer. There has never been any research showing health benefits of blocking UV light to the eyes. However, it is now impossible to buy eyeglasses that allow full-spectrum light. All of the lenses made in the last twenty years for eyeglasses are made to block UV light, even plastic lenses, which if untreated, allow full-spectrum light.

Earl Staelin, writing in the Well Being Journal, summarizes the recommendations of those who have studied light and its health effects, and recommends that individuals who must wear glasses try to get outdoors everyday for 20 to 60 minutes or more without wearing any glasses. If the weather makes this impractical, then it would be beneficial to try to function without glasses indoors under full-spectrum lighting, because the amount of UV light that strikes the retina from around the edges of glasses is insignificant compared to the large amount of light coming through the eye through the lenses. The full spectrum of daylight need not come from direct sunlight, but is available also on a cloudy day or under the shade of a tree or porch. Glass windows however, do block out UV light, so try to get out in the fresh air if at all possible.

For an especially busy person, eating your breakfast outdoors, weather permitting, may be the only option.

On days when even this is difficult, there is yet another recourse, which is distilled cod liver oil. The distillation takes out mercury and other heavy metals, which are all too prevalent in both salt and freshwater fish. Cod liver oil is high in vitamins D and A. Just 2 tablespoons a day has been found to completely eliminate psoriasis, a disease that conventional medicine only knows to suppress with steroid drugs. However, for your optimal intake, depending on your sun exposure and weight, you should really check with your naturopathic physician.

# Chapter 33
# Heart disease and diet

**Did you know . . .**

The first heart attack was reported in the medical literature only in 1912, a very recent year in all of human history. Consider that 1912 was about the time that sugar was diffusing out of the Caribbean and becoming a regular component of the western diet. However, it was many millennia after such saturated fats as lard, butter, tallow, whale blubber and other animal fat, which is available all over the world, in one form or another, had been used on a regular daily basis. So the next time the "experts" bring up the saturated fat boogeyman, but say nothing of the health-damaging effects of sugar, just think about why no one, nobody at all to the best of recorded history, had a heart attack before 1912. For any remaining confusion about the direct connection between sugar and heart disease, as well as 145 other diseases, see Nancy

Appleton's article: "146 reasons why sugar is ruining your health."[53]

**Vitamin C: superior to statins for beating heart disease**

A recent study in The American Journal of Clinical Nutrition[54] reviewed nine different studies on the subject. Their findings: "Adults who regularly take Vitamin C pills providing greater than 700 milligrams per day will experience a 25% drop in their risk for coronary heart disease.

Contrast this with a study in the Journal of the American Medical Association.[55] Their findings: "Studies have demonstrated that statins administered to individuals with risk factors for coronary heart disease (CHD) reduce CHD events. However, many of these studies were too small to assess all-cause mortality or outcomes in important subgroups. Pravastatin did *not* reduce either all-cause mortality or CHD significantly when compared with usual care in older participants." (Emphasis ours)

---

[53] Appleton, Nancy. PhD. "146 ways sugar ruins your health (with references)". Her famous article can be found on the internet at http://www.nancyappleton.com

[54] Knekt P, Ritz J, Pereira MA et al, "Antioxidant vitamins and coronary heart disease risk: a pooled analysis of 9 cohorts." American Journal of Clinical Nutrition. 2004; 80(6):1508-1520.

[55] "Major outcomes in moderately hypercholesterolemic, hypertensive patients randomized to pravastatin vs usual care: the antihypertensive and lipid-lowering treatment to prevent heart attack trial;" JAMA. 2002; 288 (23): 2998-3007.

# Chapter 34
# The world vs. the ear

What do jackhammers, rock concerts, emergency sirens and power mowers have in common? They all contribute to gradual and permanent damage of one of the most exquisitely perfect organs in our body: the ear. Not that we are born with any imperfect organs, but both the structure and function of the ear are quite magnificent.

The auricle or outer ear is so optimally sculpted that its acoustical performance is comparable to that of a concert hall. It directs sound waves from the external cacophony into the middle ear, where the waves are then amplified by the eardrum or tympanic membrane. As the eardrum vibrates, it sets into motion three tiny bones, the incus, malleus and stapes (or if you prefer the anvil, hammer and stirrups respectively) to push against the fluid inside the cochlea. This fluid then moves the hair cells of our inner ear in just such a way as to record nerve impulses. These nerve impulses are specific and varied enough that they tell your brain whether you're listening to a violin, your washing machine or the last call for dinner, as well as all the different nuances of the violin playing, if the washing machine is functioning well or half-broken, or if the last call for dinner is in a patient or frustrated tone – each transmitted by subtle and unique permutations of fluid waves.

Now, however, the music is fading out for many people. Over 28 million Americans have hearing loss ranging from mild to severe. Experts are predicting 78 million hearing loss sufferers by the year 2030.[56] Those in their fifties and sixties are experiencing the fastest decline, as the hair cells begin to show wear and tear, and as the Woodstock generation faces the music, or rather lack of it, from listening to way too loud music over the years.

The iPod generation however shows an even worse prognosis, because today's acoustic technology is so precise as to allow users to turn the volume up high without distortion. Worse still, the sound is delivered much closer to the eardrum and can cause damage faster. Some studies have found that many people's personal music is arriving at the eardrum at 115 decibels, which can cause permanent damage listening for only 28 seconds per day. Unfortunately, more than 7% of Generation Xers have damaged ears already.[57] [58]

Once hearing damage occurs it is for the most part not reversible. However, most of the current epidemic of hearing loss is completely preventable. Will the iPod generation even be able to participate in calm conversations in their middle age, or will they have to shout to each other? Will they have any conversation at all in the senior years, when they may cherish that connection with others the most?

---

[56] Noonan D. A little bit louder, please. Newsweek. June 6, 2005.
[57] Better Hearing Institute http://www.betterhearing.org.
[58] Mercola, J., D.O., A high-tech caution: taking care of your ears. Mercola.com health blog. August 15, 2005.

Well, what is an iPod listening, video game playing, high-horse-powered driving, trailblazing, double-throttle lifestyle American to do? Hmmm. Maybe it's time to slow down a little, pick the daisies and appreciate the good life, while we can still hear what's going on around us.

A good start would be to minimize use of power tools. Compare a power lawn mower, with a hand push mower, for example:

Power mower cost: $179 for a walk-behind, to $6000 for a tractor mower

Push mower cost: $39 to $179. Our $80 model is four years old and working fine.

Power mower damage to ears: high decibels, constant pitch, prolonged and frequent use – none of which is in the best interests of your hearing.

Push mower damage to ears: So quiet you can hear the wheels roll through the grass . . . fine for the ears.

Power mower calories burned: only as much as driving or slowly walking.

Push mower calories burned: 400 – 450 per hour, as much as playing tennis for the same amount of time!

Further errands after power mowing: The power mower provides too little exercise and too much noise. So now it's time to go to the gym, where you may be subjected to blaring music. You'll need to free up a lot of your weekend for this: time for power mowing, and then another hour or so for the round trip gym workout.

Further errands after push mowing: You've finished! The yard work is done, and you did it efficiently, by getting your exercise done too. Not only that, but it was all quiet – no assault on the ears.

More errands after power mowing: Get gas and oil. Tune up and repair engine. Sharpen blades.

More errands after push mowing: Sharpen blades once a year.

Yet another errand after power mowing: dispersing the grass clippings around your lawn for mulch, or more expensively, throwing those clippings away and spending extra time and money on lawn fertilizer.

Yet another errand after push mowing: You've finished! While you mowed, the grass clippings have been dispersed evenly by your push mower, for a free and effective fertilizer on your lawn.

People with immense lawns may not be able to replace their power mowing easily. However, for a low investment, you can start to cut some of the grass with a push mower for a quiet, fresh air workout.

Here are other alternatives to the noisy, energy-gobbling appliances around our homes:

- hanging clothes out to dry, just takes a few minutes.
- using a hand-cranked food grater/processor, less than a minute.
- hand washing the dishes, a good chore for the kids or for the spouse who does not have the cooking duties
- Letting your hair air-dry. (A hair dryer is a huge 14 watts and quite a noisy appliance to have next to your ear.)

Other quiet activities that are becoming a lost art:

- reading and writing
- prayer or meditation
- gardening
- yoga
- hiking or early morning mall-walking or snowshoeing or cross-country skiing
- bird watching
- fishing
- plant/flower/rock identification
- knitting and other fine needle arts
- other art, such as whittling, sculpture and painting

Social activities that are fairly quiet include the following:

- Spiritual/religious gatherings
- Volunteering in a Montessori classroom (pretty quiet, self-directed work)
- Continuing education, poetry readings, conferences (not silent, but not blaring either)
- Last but not least, the almost forgotten art of reading aloud from works of classic literature to the whole family. One family reads Charles Dickens' *A Christmas Carol* out loud (taking turns) every Christmas season. What a wonderful way to celebrate a holiday, introduce younger children to the classics, enhance the education of older children, not to mention their SAT English scores, stretch kids' attention span, entertain adults, foster appreciation, participation and familiarity with great literature in every family member, and actually (horrors!) involve the parents and children in the same activity in the same room at the same time, while enjoying each others' company. This lost art of reading aloud can expanded to gatherings of multiple families and/or neighbors, and can include potluck or snacks. Not a silent activity, but not ear-threatening either.

Of course, hearing aids are becoming technically better, smaller and even implantable. But we all know the most natural treatment for any malady: prevention. So turning down the volume, avoiding loud theaters, choosing hand tools over power tools when practical, and finding quiet activities with your family, friends or alone can all go a long way toward preserving two of your greatest instruments of social interaction and appreciation of the good life: your two ears.

# Chapter 35
# Earache at Midnight: What do you do?

Parents of young children often notice that children's earaches do not follow doctors' office hours. Small children can experience such intense pain in the ears that it wakes them out of deep sleep.

When this happens there are a number of naturopathic treatments that can be used by parents to bring prompt relief.

## Apply a poultice

Application of warmth behind the ear can be used to mobilize the post-auricular lymph chain and vasculature and to draw congestion away from the inflamed area of the middle ear. To do this, heat half of an onion in a toaster oven for a few minutes, until it is warm but not intolerably hot when applied to your own ear or inner forearm for several seconds. Wrap the onion in cheesecloth or thin dishcloth, and apply the largest side (the cut side, for maximum surface area) to the area just behind the ear. If the child feels that the poultice is still too hot, have her hold it as close as she can tolerate while it cools. As she moves it toward her skin, give her enough pillows to prop her arm comfortably while she holds the poultice.

A variation on this that has also shown quick results is to score with a knife the cut surface of the onion, just making a checkerboard of parallel cuts about ¼" deep. This is to allow the strong juice of the onion (onion as botanical medicine, *Allium cepa*) to diffuse. Without baking it, you can place the onion directly on the ear.

**Acupressure**

There are a number of acupuncture points, close to and away from the ear, that provide relief from earache. Start on the wrist. From the wrist crease at the back of the hand, measure two of the child's (not your) thumbwidths up the arm, toward the elbow. Pressing this point, known as Sanjiao 5, you will feel the end of the groove between the two long bones of the forearm. Press and massage this point on both wrists. One child told me that while I pressed this point, the "owie" went away completely just then. Also press the fleshy mound on the back of the hand where the base of the thumb meets the hand. Press and manipulate this point on both sides.

Points near the ear also help. Find the point on the neck at the bottom of the earlobe. Press and manipulate this point on both sides. Then on the front of the ear there are a series of points along the vertical line where the ear meets the face. If the child tolerates it press and massage along this line on each side.

**Consider the cause**

According to the New England Journal of Medicine, acute ear infection in children, or otitis media, is most commonly caused by viruses,[59] yet the standard therapy in pediatric practice remains antibiotics, a useless treatment for viral infections. Another study found no benefit from decongestants, another common treatment.[60] A study reported in the Journal of the American Medical Association found that many times tympanostomy tubes or ear tubes were placed for inappropriate or equivocal indications.[61] It has also been found that the placing of ear tubes did not improve long-term outcomes.[62]

With a view toward natural treatment, self-limiting viral diseases, such as the majority of ear infections, are treated by supporting the immune system. To this end, bioflavonoids, such as those found in berries may be an especially appropriate and tasty medicine for the ill child. Garlic may be used for anti-viral effects. Other botanical and nutritional interventions would be recommended by a naturopathic physician with consideration of the child's metabolic type and medical and family history. A naturopathic physician would also consider the particular presentation of the individual patient's case as a main determinant of what treatment to offer. The unusual complications of otitis media, such as mastoiditis, labyrinthitis, meningitis or brain abscess, do require emergency treatment.

Also the removal of irritants and allergens should be a priority. Second hand cigarette smoke contributes to incidence of otitis media. Consumption of dairy products, particularly pasteurized dairy is a culprit for many children. Other food items in the diet

---

[59] Heikkinen, New England Journal of Medicine, 1999.
[60] Buchanan, Archives of pediatric and Adolescent Medicine, 1999.
[61] Kleinman, Journal of the American Medical Association, 1994.
[62] Paradise, New England Journal of Medicine, 2001.

that seem to be followed by symptoms should be eliminated, at least until symptoms disappear.

## The Long Term View

The goal for treatment should be to eliminate the susceptibility of the individual to repeated attacks or infections. Parents may wish to consult with a naturopathic physician, which you can find at www.naturopathic.org, or other qualified health care provider. Such a doctor can make a thorough and professional evaluation of the child's past medical history, family medical history, environmental challenges, diet, and other factors and identify likely problems and solutions. Many naturopaths practice homeopathy, which in the hands of an experienced homeopath, can eliminate not only the disease but the susceptibility to recurrence of the disease. If acupuncture is employed, the most effective and complete point prescription for the patient may be determined by a qualified professional. Other natural medicine, such as hydrotherapy and cranio-sacral manipulation may also be appropriately employed to rid a child of ear infections.

# Chapter 36
# Carsick or seasick?
# Ancient Chinese medicine can help

Try pressing Pericardium 6 whenever you find yourself in the miserable sloshing of endless ocean waves or as a passenger being thrown back and forth on a winding road in the mountains with many hairpin turns.

Pericardium 6 may be found from the center of your wrist crease on the palm side, two thumb-widths up (toward the heart). Once you've located that general area, press and massage as needed for relief during your journey.

This point is quite useful for nausea and vomiting generally, as well as travel sickness and morning sickness in pregnancy. In fact, some drugstores sell a bracelet or wrist band which can be worn on a boat or in a car that will provide continual stimulation to the point Pericardium 6 for relief of motion sickness.

# Chapter 37
# Heartburn relief from acupressure

A study out of Australia last month has confirmed what traditional Chinese medicine has taught for millenia: to relieve heartburn, an acupuncture point on the wrist may be pressed – not necessarily needled, for those who don't particularly enjoy being poked with pointy metal objects.

The study found that the abnormal laxity of the lower esophageal sphincter (LES), which is what allows stomach acids to back up and "burn" the esophagus, is normalized by pressure on the Neiguan, or Pericardium 6, point. It was found that the stimulation of Pericardium 6 reduced laxity or excessive relaxations of the sphincter by 40 percent.

According to traditional Chinese medicine, acupuncture points on the skin are aligned with internal pathways or meridians that run through the inside of the body, conducting energy. Stimulation of the points may take the form of simply pressing with one's finger, needle stimulation, or stimulation with electricity, heat, light or colored light.

The Director of the study was cautious however, and said, "It is too soon to recommend acupuncture for battling heartburn. There is no justification at this stage for heartburn sufferers to rush out and receive acupoint stimulation treatment."

We agree with part of what Dr. Holloway said: No need to "rush out." In fact, you can stimulate this point in the privacy of your own home, in fact right now. Place either hand in front of you, palm up. Using your other thumb, measure two thumb widths up from the middle of your wrist crease palm side, in the direction of the elbow crease. Now locate the point two thumbwidths up from the middle of your wrist crease. That is Pericardium 6. or Neiguan, a very useful point which we have written about in the last chapter. Heartburn sufferers may want to stimulate this point following a meal, a little before the time they would normally feel symptoms of heartburn. You may find a heartburn sufferer very grateful to you if you let them know about Pericardium 6.

Acupuncture is actually a complete system of medicine, with very powerful results. Naturopathic physicians throughout Arizona and a number of other states are trained in traditional Chinese medicine and use acupuncture or acupressure with patients whom think they could benefit and may be interested in that kind of treatment.

# Chapter 38
# Fever: ally or enemy?

"Give me a fever, and I can cure any illness" -- *Hippocrates*

Many parents consider a fever to be something dangerous in itself. There are parents who are so afraid of fever that if their child's temperature rises to 100° or 101° F, they give their child a liver toxin such as acetaminophen or the gut-scraping ibuprofen. Worse yet, there are parents who have given their children aspirin at first sign of fever, which is an extremely dangerous risk for the life-threatening Reye's Disease. How did fever come to be seen as such a dangerous condition that we put our child's wellbeing at risk in order to suppress temperature?

Let's first consider the functions of fever and how it works:

The two functions of fever are:

1) to stimulate the immune system, as described below, and

2) to create an inhospitable environment for invading organisms. That is, to turn up the heat high enough that the invading microbes cannot live.

When almost any kind of microbe invades the body, it is eaten alive by the first line of defense: macrophages (literally, "big eaters"). Macrophages then recruit other immune system cells and make Interleukin One (IL-1). IL-1 is one of several endogenous pyrogens, which means that it is something that is a part of your body that gives the signal to raise temperature.

So here's how a fever is made: IL-1, along with other pyrogens and proteins is released into the blood, and makes its way up to the hypothalamus in your brain. Now the hypothalamus is that little perfectionist part of us that says the temperature must be just 98.6°, and our hormones must be maintained just right, at certain more or less fixed quantities in the bloodstream. So when the picky hypothalamus gets the IL-1 signal, it now knows that 98.6° just isn't enough anymore. Now we've got the highly unusual circumstance of many invading pathogens, and in extraordinary times like these, the temperature must be raised a few degrees if we're going to get rid of that bug and keep the body healthy. So the hypothalamus makes another biochemical, PGE-2. PGE-2 then increases the body temperature set point, to say 101° or 102° F, or wherever it's determined by the hypothalamus to be sufficient for protecting the body from the bug.

So how does the body actually raise its temperature, once the hypothalamus has determined that it's necessary to do so? If we're still healthy and youthful enough to accomplish everything up to this point, then our heat generating mechanisms include the following: shivering, the hormone TRH and vasoconstriction. Another one is piloerection, or raising the small hairs, which is involved with suppressed sweat. Sweat is a cooling mechanism, so we now have heat being generated, but not much is being lost.

What a fantastic synergy we have of self-healing mechanisms in our bodies – a veritable symphony of coordinated responses involved with fever.

Now that we have a raging fever, let's look at the benefits of it:

- more antibodies produced – cells trained to specifically attack the exact type of invader that your body is presently suffering from – more specific to that bug than any pharmaceutical;

- more white blood cells (the good guys) produced, more of them circulating and mobile and armed to fight off the invading bugs, and specific to the general category of invader;

- more interferon produced (another immune system component, which blocks spread of viruses to healthy cells);

- walling off of iron, which bacteria feed on;

- increased temperature, which directly kills microbes. (Most bacteria and viruses actually grow better at temperatures lower than the human body – which is why they like our cool noses in the winter.) Parents, it's not your kids needing fever-reducing drugs; it's the germs!

Naturopathic treatment is to support a fever, unless it rises too high or too quickly. A fever of 102° to 103° degrees Fahrenheit is considered optimal for best effect against microbes and for healing the body the most effectively. Supporting a fever means to work with it. For example, one effect of fever is to slow down peristalsis, which is movement of food through the gut. So to support fever, naturopathic physicians recommend either fasting or minimal food, such as broths and water till the fever breaks. Fever is also best supported with rest. Even when the child or other patient may seem sleepy on the outside, the body is working quite hard to carry out all the functions described above. Exercise and activity both distract body energy from these vitally important immune system processes. Naturopaths look at acute disease as the body's attempt to cure. Therefore, support the body's defenses; don't suppress them.

Naturopathic physicians consider that fear of symptoms is like a fear of your car's engine light. To suppress a fever is like asking your mechanic to disconnect the engine light, rather than asking him to identify and fix the problem that caused the light to come on in the first place. Parents should ask themselves how they can approach their children's symptoms as logically as they approach their cars: do we really want to suppress our warning signals? In the case of fever, the warning signal is much more of an aid to conquering illness, rather than a source of damage in itself.

Some exceptions to letting a fever run its course are listed below. Medical attention is warranted for fever in the following circumstances:

- Infants less than 1 month old, with a temperature greater than 100.4° F. Seek care right away for fever in this age group. While waiting for care, breastfeed as often as the baby desires. The mother's milk has antibodies made right at the breast as it encounters pathogens in the baby's mouth.

- Infants from 1 month to 3 months old, with a temperature greater than 100.4°, if they appear ill. Again, breastfeed on demand while waiting for care.

- Children between 3 months and 36 months, with a temperature above 102.2°, if they appear ill.

- Anyone with a temperature over 104.5° F.

For children not in the above categories, bed rest and fluids will support the fever and allow it to do the job that your child needs it to do.

# Chapter 39
# Fast help for a bad back

Some days you may find yourself too busy to make it out for a back adjustment. If there were something you could do yourself, you could get out of misery and rescue the day.

It must be acknowledged first that there are certain back aches that constitute medical emergencies, and must be imaged right away, either with x-ray, CT or MRI. The following types of backache must be investigated immediately, and if you have any of these, you need to get medical attention. For example, a backache that begins for no particular reason, without trauma or strain, or one that is accompanied by either incontinence or loss of sensation anywhere in the body. Also, there are some abdominal conditions that may result in backache and need to be investigated. These include pancreatitis or gallstones, which often radiate to various parts of the back. Also, if there are metastases from cancer elsewhere in the body there may be resulting back pain.

If, however, your backache is old and familiar, or from known injury or muscle strain, then you probably have a chronic or acute musculoskeletal condition that can be helped by some of the following at-home interventions.

**How to use a hot shower**

Once you figure out which muscles are most sore you can contract and relax them under the warm water of the shower. Contract for a slow count of 5, and relax for a slow count of five, while staying in the same position. Repeat this at least 3 times. You can also do this out of the shower, but the heat of the shower water will give you even more effective muscle relaxation, so that your aching muscles can more easily release the spasms that are causing you pain.

**How to use acupressure**

For lower back pain, reach down and press the point that is in the middle of the crease in back of your knee. Press on both knees, rubbing and massaging that point, until you work out any sharp discomfort you may find there, or for a minute at least.

Here are another couple of points for low back pain: On the back of your hand, look halfway between your knuckles and your wrist crease. Along this line, press the points in between the metacarpal bones (the long straight bones that run from your wrist to your knuckles).

For shoulder and neck pain, here is a different point. Make a loose fist and look at your little finger and the side of your hand. See the crease that points to your knuckle? At the end of that crease, near the knuckle, press and knead that point.

Having acupuncture done by your acupuncturist or naturopathic doctor is more effective, because only an L.Ac or ND can give you an individual diagnosis and a needling and herb treatment that is specific for the type of back pain and general health condition that you have. Your naturopathic physician can order any imaging or blood work that may be necessary to correctly diagnose your back pain. However, in a pinch, the acupressure points mentioned above can help relieve some of the misery.

## Ergonomics

Ergonomically designed furniture is not one size fits all. If your desk chair or other chair where you do most of your sedentary work is not comfortable, then it is not appropriate for you. Bring in the cushions or pillows necessary to get your back into a position of ease. Keep adjusting as needed until the ache is minimized or gone. This also encourages the release of muscle spasm.

## Exercise

No discussion of back pain is complete without acknowledging an unavoidable truth: the nerves surrounding the bones and muscles of your back are only going to be as tolerable to you as the muscles that support that whole architecture. And the only way to keep those muscles lifting what they are supposed to lift is by strengthening them with exercise. Unlike the exercise described above for releasing a muscle spasm, the exercises below are long-term strengthening exercises, which you should incorporate into your workout. (Of course, you have a workout. All healthy people do! If you don't, okay then, you can start today. No not tomorrow. Today.)

Depending on which type of low back pain you have, one of the following exercises will be more useful to you than the other. Try both for best effect:

Lie on your back, and lift both feet a few inches up from the floor. Hold for a count of ten, then lower feet to floor. Repeat 3 times. This will also exercise your abdominal muscles as well as some back muscles.

To do the other exercise, roll onto your abdomen. Bring your head and upper body up, resting on your elbows. Tighten your back muscles for a count of ten. Relax for a few seconds. Repeat 3 times.

**Pregnant women and heart disease patients should consult their physician before beginning these or other exercises. If these or other exercises are contraindicated for you, then yoga may be a more appropriate alternative.**

# Chapter 40
# Counterstrain for Sore Muscles

There is a technique that is gentle, easy to perform and effective for sore muscles. This short summary is borrowed from traditional osteopathy, but can be used by anyone. Run your fingers along the length of your sore muscle. For example, if the back and side of your neck is sore, run your fingers from behind your ear down to the top of your shoulder. This step is so that you can know and picture in your mind which muscle you will be shortening. Try to locate and memorize the exact location of the most sore spot along the sore muscle.

Now, trying not to use that muscle at all, with both hands, place yourself in such a position that the sore muscle is as short as possible (the opposite of stretching that muscle). For example, if the right side of your neck is sore, you will position your head to the right. You may need to lie down or use furniture as a prop to be able to keep this muscle completely relaxed. You can shorten the muscle by basically curling yourself around it. Still not using the sore muscle, use your hands or prop to maintain yourself in the same position to keep the sore muscle shortened. Make slight adjustments (forward, back, left, right, etc.) until the point that was sore now feels the best possible. Now hold that position for 90 seconds, again not using or tensing the sore muscle, just placing yourself in position with your hands.

At the end of 90 seconds use only your hands to gently reposition yourself to normal. Now press the sore point again. If it is 70% improved or better, you have done good Counterstrain. It may take a whole day to really feel improved.

The way Counterstrain works is that it relaxes the muscle sufficiently to allow a spasm or tightness in the muscle to loosen by itself. If you get some relief but not enough, try it again in a slightly modified position. You have only 90 seconds to lose.

# Chapter 41
# Long life, from your shins

In traditional Chinese Medicine, qi (pronounced "chee") is the source of your energy and vitality. Qi may often appear to be lacking especially in adults. One traditional Chinese recommendation for long life is to press the acupuncture point known as "Stomach 36" every day, making a habit of it. Stomach 36 may be found by first locating the dimple on the outside of your bent knee. You will find it surrounded by three bones (your femur, tibia and patella). Now measure one of your own hand widths (must be *your own* hand width) down the shin. Press on the point one hand width down from the dimple. You should be pressing in the top of the groove between the shafts of the tibia and fibula. If a picture of the point would help, go to:

http://www.acuxo.blogspot.com

and locate Stomach 36 from the pull-down menus.

# Chapter 42
# Why tonic herbs are so important: Rosemary, for example

Rosemary is often used as an elder tonic, because of its three principle properties: It is a mild anti-depressant. It is a memory tonic. And it is a circulatory stimulant (which probably is what results in the other two properties.) For those with low blood pressure, the circulatory stimulation is just enough to raise blood pressure toward or into the normal range. For those with hypertension who wish to take rosemary, it is advisable to monitor blood pressure daily and discontinue rosemary in case blood pressure rises.

The circulatory stimulation of rosemary is also effective topically, and is often used as a poultice for areas of poor circulation. Rosemary enhances perfusion to the brain. Ancient Romans and Greeks wore wreaths of rosemary on their heads to enhance memory while studying, and it is still burned today in Greek students' homes during their study time.

Rosemary also has sesquiterpenes, which are secreted by the plant to fend off insects. These chemicals also have anti-fungal and anti-bacterial effects. From medieval times to World War II, rosemary branches were burned in sick rooms to disinfect the air.

Spanish Christians called rosemary "the holy herb" because of the legend that Mary draped her cloak over a rosemary bush during their flight to Egypt, which turned the blossoms from white to blue, and according to a number of references later became the source of the popular name "Rose of Mary."[63]

---

[63] See also http://www.botanical.com/botanical/mgmh/r/rosema17.html

# Chapter 43
# Chronic Inflammation Has a High Price: Don't pay it!

When you get an acute infection or injury, your body gets inflamed for a while, sending in repair teams of white blood cells, extra blood, fibroblasts and other anabolic factors to produce the heat, swelling, redness, pain and sometimes discharge that will eventually cure the problem, and return you to normal. But sometimes inflammation does not go away. When it stays with you chronically, it can cause a number of diseases, including cancer and heart disease.

Chronic inflammation starts with a stressor. This can include a long-term infection with insufficient immune response to get rid of it, excess free radicals causing oxidative damage, high blood insulin levels, an excess of arachidonic acid or other imbalance in proportion of fatty acids, and even lack of sleep. As a result, you get a buildup of the wrong prostaglandins (PG2)[64] and the wrong cytokines[65] (interleukin 6 or IL 6).

Avoidance is the best strategy for such a subtle and subclinical process as chronic inflammation. That includes sufficient sleep, eating low insulinemic foods such as lots of vegetables and moderate quantities of other whole foods, with avoidance of refined carbohydrates. This strategy will in turn stimulate your immune system to discourage long term infections from hanging around. Also, supplementing with omega-3 fatty acids, such as fish oil or flax oil will divert the inflammatory pathway away from the most damaging results. Avoidance of free radicals can be a little trickier, because there are various forms of radiation all around us. In addition to avoiding extreme or excessive exposure, think of Vitamins C and E as powerful anti-oxidant shields that protect you from free radicals. Just remember when supplementing that Vitamin C is water soluble and goes through your body quickly, while Vitamin E is fat soluble, which makes it take a while longer.

---

[64] Prostaglandins are biochemicals that we make from fatty acids in our cell membranes. Their functions vary widely. Some prostaglandins contribute to inflammatory conditions throughout the body. Others raise body temperature. Others can raise or lower blood pressure. Still others can stimulate contractions of the womb that lead to childbirth.

[65] Cytokines are biochemicals that are made by some cells to influence the actions of other cells. In the case of the interleukins, they are produced by the leukocytes or white blood cells, which become more numerous and active during infections.

# Chapter 44
# The toxic bucket

> " We are conducting a vast toxicologic experiment, and we are using our children as the experimental animals." – Dr. Philip Landrigan, Chairman, Preventive Medicine, Mt. Sinai School of Medicine

> "With chemicals, it's shoot first and ask questions later." – Al Meyerhoff, former attorney for the Natural Resources Defense Council

> "Years of documents have shown that they knew they were hurting people, much like the tobacco industry." – Sandy Buchanan, Executive Director, Ohio Citizen Action

> "Historians don't like to use broad political term like 'cover-up', but there's really no other term that you can use for this." – Prof. Gerald Markowitz, Ph.D., John Jay College.

The above quotes are taken from a documentary entitled "Trade Secrets: a Moyers Report," in which Bill Moyers examined the various trails of industrial effluent through our air, water and food, and how these trails terminate in our bones, our fat cells, our brains, our internal organs.

Chemicals are ubiquitous and increasingly present in our homes, cars and even our food. Thousands of new synthetic chemicals come into manufactured consumer products every year with no safety testing or public approval process. More than 80,000 new chemicals have been in circulation in consumer products since the rise of the petrochemical industry. Through our lungs, skin and GI tract, we are soaking up chemicals that we'd be hard-pressed to spell or pronounce, if we could even find out what they were. Human fat tissue sampled in the United States has shown 700 chemical contaminants that have not even been chemically identified.[66] A Mt. Sinai School of Medicine study found that each of nine volunteers averaged 91 chemical compounds in the blood and urine.[67] Of the 167 chemicals discovered among the volunteers tested, 94 are toxic to the brain or nervous system, 76 are carcinogenic and 79 are linked to birth defects. The volunteers

[66] Onstot, J. et al. "Characterization of HRCG/MS unidentified peaks from the analysis of human adipose tissue." Vol 1. Technical Approach, US EPA Office of Toxic Substances (560/8-87-002a); 1987.

[67] See full report with references at http://www.ewg.org.

tested do not work with chemicals on the job, nor do they live close to an industrial facility. Rather, they represent the average body burden of an ordinary American citizen. Furthermore, chemicals that are foreign to the body, or xenobiotics (*xeno* = foreign or not naturally occurring) tend to accumulate in the tissues over time. Worse, children, playing on the floor and breathing more air than adults, acquire chemical body burdens faster than adults.

This is not simply a minor disruption to optimal health. According to the World Health Organization (WHO), air pollution causes 2.7 million deaths annually. And the EPA estimates that there has been no "clean air" in the United States for over *25 years.* Even relatively pristine areas are not immune, because global air currents carry pesticides from the heavily agricultural tropical regions even as far as the polar regions, where cool air sinks them to ground level. This has given the Inuit a very high body burden of chemicals, despite their remote existence in mostly far Northern wilderness areas.

But as bad as that is, indoor air pollution is even worse. The formaldehyde and other solvents leaking out of our walls, furniture and especially carpets keep many, perhaps most of us, in a limbo between good health and vague malaise. According to a study in Effective Clinical Practice in April 1999, three out of four Americans has a diagnosable chronic condition.[68]

Against this bleak and despairing scenario, the emerging field of Environmental Medicine, a specialty within naturopathic medicine, is offering a means for people to reduce their total body burden of heavy metals and synthetic chemicals. Patients with

[68] Schwartz, L. et al., "Changing disease definitions: implications for disease prevalence: Analysis of the Third National Health and Nutrition Evaluation Survey, 1988-1994." *Effective Clinical Practice.* March/April 1999.

conditions that have completely stumped conventional doctors, conditions such as fibromyalgia, chronic fatigue, lupus, asthma, multiple sclerosis and migraines, are now finding relief and reversal of symptoms through the various cleansing procedures employed in environmental medicine.

Dr. Walter Crinnion, a naturopathic medical doctor and one of the pioneers in the emerging field of environmental medicine, prefers to use the term "cleanse" rather than "detoxify," because our enormous bodily burden of xenobiotics has so thoroughly confused the normal detoxification processes of the liver, that the liver can make some chemicals even more dangerous in the attempt to detoxify. Not having either evolved or been created to process these strange substances, the liver quite literally does not know what to do with them, and in breaking them down can liberate even more dangerous components. Therefore, the first goal of environmental medicine is "avoidance," simply avoiding exposure to chemical toxins. Failing that, as constantly happens, the next goal of environmental medicine, is to grab the macromolecule, before it is broken down, and haul it out of the body before it can do much harm.

However, most patients don't begin to seek help from environmental medical specialists until years of bombardment with toxic chemicals has taken a huge toll on their health. So what we are then dealing with in many cases are the metabolites, or bodily-derived chemicals, from the original pollutants. The body's unfamiliarity with synthetic chemicals sometimes prevents it from processing them at all, and they are simply stored in fat cells, as the ultimate repository of strange items. As a result, overweight people have even more of a body burden than the rest of us.

Some of the most prevalent chemicals are the dioxins that are common in pesticides, the volatile and semi-volatile compounds such as styrene, xylene, etc. that are commonly used in manufacturing, chlorinated compounds, such as DDT and PCBs, which are accumulating not only in the foods that they are sprayed on, but all the way up the food chain, becoming ever more concentrated on the way up, including in the big game fish of the Atlantic. Heavy metals are also accumulating in our oceans and the fish there. These are some of the xenobiotics that appear to be present in everyone.

Some of the cleansing processes involve coaxing fat –bound substances away from fat cells. Since the brain is 60% fat, it is a primary storage site of these chemicals. Mercury is very strongly attracted to fat, which is much of the reason why children poisoned with mercury, which is still in many vaccines and amalgam dental fillings, show autistic and hyperactive symptoms primarily. Mercury is also a neurotoxin, which means it is a slow poison to the brain. It is also known to be associated with Alzheimers Disease.

The majority of xenobiotics undergo metabolic changes, known as biotransformation, in which fat-soluble compounds are converted into water-soluble compounds, which allows them to be excreted by the body. For these compounds, Dr. Crinnion's strategy is to help this excretion along, both by assisting the normal cleansing processes in the liver, and by removing obstacles to those processes introduced by other xenobiotics. Many pharmaceuticals act as obstacles to the liver's cleansing process. Also, high sugar consumption as well as protein deprivation are both obstacles to optimal cleansing function of the liver. Various vitamin, mineral and amino acid deficiencies also inhibit the liver from effective cleansing.

So what is the "toxic bucket"? It is the human body, descended from eons of pure-air breathing, whole-food eating, clean-water drinking ancestors, who lived in perfect biochemical harmony with their earth. But the toxic bucket is really the modern human body, descended from that beautiful harmonious existence, now tarnished and contaminated with chemicals that enter continually through every orifice and pore.

The assault on our bodies from the huge numbers of synthetic chemicals in our environment is a life-threatening challenge for a planet and its inhabitants that are not acclimated to such substances. Thus the most effective therapeutic approach for the chemical-laden patient involves several steps: avoidance of further exposure to whatever extent possible, dietary changes and cleansing procedures. Naturopathic physicians (Naturopathic Doctors (NDs) and Naturopathic Medical Doctors (NMDs)) are trained during four years of naturopathic medical school in the procedures necessary to help patients keep their "bucket" of toxic substances as empty as possible, and to help the cleansed body function as well as possible. The directory of naturopathic physicians on the website of the American Association of Naturopathic Physicians, which is the largest database of naturopathic physicians in the U.S., www.naturopathic.org, is where U.S. residents can find a local naturopathic physician.

# Chapter 45
# The newborn's toxic burden

In the months leading up to a baby's birth, the umbilical cord carries blood back and forth between the fetus and the placenta - where oxygen and nutrients are picked up by the blood for delivery to the developing baby.

Although it has been known that there are some substances harmful to a developing fetus which readily cross the placenta blood barrier; alcohol[69] being a prime example, for a long time it was thought that the placenta acted as a rather efficient "filter" removing the majority of toxins from the fetal blood supply thereby allowing it to develop unaffected by harmful substances. In fact, any maternal alcohol during the peri-conceptual period,

[69] Center for Disease Control. Alcohol and Public Health" General alcohol information. http://www.cdc.gov/alcohol

which is considered three months before and three months after conception, may result in a *six-fold* increase in Sudden Infant Death Syndrome (SIDS) in the newborn.[70]

Now a study conducted by the Environmental Working Group (www.ewg.org) and Commonweal (www.commonweal.org), has shown that the placenta is not as efficient a filter as was once thought. Using cord blood taken from 10 U.S. babies born between August and September 2004, tests were conducted in an attempt to detect some 260 different chemicals. Essentially all of the chemicals tested for were found in the cord blood samples including pesticides, consumer product ingredients (perfluorinated chemicals associated with products like Teflon, Scotchgard, carpet protectors and food wraps), and waste products produced by burning both coal and gasoline. This joint study is the first reported detection of over 200 of the chemicals in cord blood.

These findings are of particular concern for a number of reasons:

1. In a developing child, and particularly in the fetus, chemical exposure is greater on a pound-for-pound basis than for an adult.
2. An immature, porous blood-brain barrier allows greater chemical exposures to the brain - even into teenage years.
3. A baby's organs and systems are rapidly developing. This makes them more vulnerable to damage from chemical exposures.
4. Systems such as the liver that remove toxins from the body are not yet fully developed in infants and children.
5. A longer anticipated remaining life span of a child (when compared to an adult) allows more time for the negative effects of chemical exposure to arise.

---

[70] Ibid.

Today there are approximately 75,000 chemical compounds in use in the United States. In addition - an average of 7 new chemicals are introduced into use every day. The vast majority of these chemicals are used with little or no testing with regard to the long-term effect they have on our health. This is in spite of evidence that chemical exposures can and do have much more significant effects on the very young and yet to be born as evidenced by the mercury poisoning disaster of the 1950s in Minamata Japan[71] and how in the case of DES[72] the way our genes may even be re-programmed in ways that are both undesirable and lasting ways.

Couples planning to start a family in the near future are increasingly taking the strategy of consulting with an environmental medical specialist to test for chemical and heavy metal exposure. These are then chelated out of both prior to attempting conception, in order to give the children a better non-toxic start to their lives. Naturopathic doctors study environmental medicine, with some specializing more than others

[71] Minamata was a fishing village that suffered such a severe and dramatic onslaught of industrial pollution, especially mercury poisoning in the 1950's, that the number of victims has been climbing steadily ever since. The Chisso company began to make acetaldehyde near Minamata Bay, and effluent from the process left the baywater, then the fish – a major part of the Japanese diet – so polluted with mercury that they were often found belly-up in the water. Then moving up the food chain, cats began to behave bizarrely and drowned themselves in the Bay, a phenomenon known as "the cat suicides" and finally people began to have tremors, stumbling, sudden shouting, diminished hearing and comprehension, with a steadily climbing death rate. It is now estimated that there are 10,000 victims, plus another 3,000 dead from Minamata Disease.

[72] DES or diethylstilbestrol is a synthetic estrogen that was prescribed to pregnant women in order to prevent complications of pregnancy from 1938 to 1971. However, the complications are affecting the next two generations. Daughters of women who were given DES have had increased risk of breast cancer and adenocarcinoma of the cervix and vagina. Children and grandchildren of both sexes are at somewhat increased risk of genital abnormalities and rare cancers.

in this area. One of the leaders in environmental medicine is Dr. Walter Crinnion. For further information on environmental medicine please see Dr. Doris Rapp's books: *Our Toxic World* and *Is This Your Child's World?*

See the Environmental Working Group site, www.ewg.org, for the full report – *BodyBurden: The Pollution in Newborns.* See also the Naturopathyworks page on Environmental Medicine at www.natureworksbest.com/naturopathy-works/toxic-bucket.

# Chapter 46
# Non-toxic bath products

More than one-third of all personal care products contain at least one ingredient linked to cancer, according to the non-partisan, non-profit Environmental Working Group (EWG).

The biggest problem is that the cosmetics industry has always stayed under the radar of regulation. The Food and Drug Administration has no mandate to safety-test cosmetics. The extent of the FDA policy in the area is that "manufacturers may use any ingredient or raw material, except for color additives and a few prohibited substances, to market a product without a government review or approval."

There is a self-policing Cosmetic Ingredient Review (CIR) panel, which is an industry-funded panel of seven scientists and physicians. They study potentially hazardous ingredients and make non-binding recommendations. Yet only 11% of the 10,500 ingredients in cosmetics have been evaluated for safety according to the EWG.

As far as actual cause and effect, little is known, and suspected connections are very difficult to prove. Cancer rates continue to rise, yet of the tens of thousands of synthetic chemicals in our environment, less than one percent of these are well-known regarding their health effects. The sheer numbers and proximity of these chemicals defy any attempt to sort out the good from the bad.

Bath products, soaps and cosmetics are particularly troublesome, because we absorb more toxins from what we breathe and what contacts our skin than even by eating and drinking.

Here are some things we do know about common bath products:

**Parabens** (Methylparaben, propylparaben, etc.) are the most common preservatives for personal care products in the U.S. They are in shampoos, soaps, toothpastes, deodorants, and eye, ear and nose drops, among many other products. (They are also present in such prepared foods as mayonnaise, mustard, jams and jellies, salad dressings, soft drinks, baked goods and candy.) Water is the only ingredient used more frequently. Whether parabens are harmful or not is a tough question and it all depends on whom you ask. Intense industry pressure in the United States has accomplished the predictable whitewash from paid "researchers." However, scientists in other countries have found that parabens affect the body much the same way as estrogens. In males and females this can cause diminished muscle mass and extra fat storing, as well as gynecomastia (breast growth) in males. Some studies have found intact parabens in human breast tumors, as well as contributing factors from parabens in the growth of the tumors. (Routledge, et al. 1998)

A study from the Journal of Toxicology found that the concentration of parabens in human breast tumors was found to be 20.6 +/- 4.2 ng per gram of tissue. Methylparaben was present at the highest level (12.8 +/- 2.2 ng per gram of tissue).[73]

Ethyl alcohol is another ingredient used as a solvent in large proportion in many personal care products. It does not only serve to mix other ingredients during manufacture, but is also a solvent when it hits your skin. Its drying effect makes its presence in such products as "moisturizing" skin lotions something of a Trojan Horse. The result is you get drier than when you started, and are tempted to keep reapplying, and keep buying, the "moisturizing" lotion.

## Healthier alternatives

Our basic advice is to stay away from new molecules as much as possible, simply as a general principle to avoid unnecessary cancer risks.

### 1) Deodorant

Did you know that instead of commercial deodorant, you can have a completely effective, all-day deodorant, that will stay with you

---

[73] Darbre PD, Aljarrah A, Miller WR, Coldham NG, Sauer MJ, Pope GS. Concentrations of parabens in human breast tumours. Journal of Toxicology. Division of Cell and Molecular Biology, School of Animal and Microbial Sciences, University of Reading, Reading RG6 6AJ, UK. p.d.dabre@reading.ac.uk

through the gym, a mile-run and more for the price of baking soda?

Bring a small container of baking soda to your bathroom sink. Take a pinch of baking soda in one hand. Drop several drops of water on it. The exact proportion doesn't matter at all. Rub your hands together, then rub each hand lightly on the opposite underarm. You will be amazed at how effective baking soda is as a deodorant. It can be irritating right after shaving though, so try to separate the two by using baking soda on different days than shaving or different times of the day.

**2) Shampoo**

At almost any health food store you will find Dr. Bronner's Pure Castile Soap. This is at least a clean non-chemical soap that you can use for both shampoo and body wash. If you want to enrich it for a hair-growth stimulating mixture, pour a few tablespoons of rosemary oil into the shampoo, and shake lightly just to combine. Because rosemary oil can be expensive, I make my own. Rosemary is sold at many nurseries and neighborhood plant shops especially around Christmas when it is usually pruned to a Christmas tree shape. Once you get your rosemary bush to a robust size, you can prune it lightly. Stuff a glass jar full with the rinsed and dried rosemary cuttings, and pour in extra virgin olive oil to completely cover. Now put it in a dark place, and forget about it for six weeks. At the end you will have a lovely rosemary oil infusion, which you can then add to the Dr. Bronner's liquid soap.

**3) Soaps**

Dr. Bronner also makes hard soaps with no synthetic ingredients, available at health food stores. So does Hugo Saavedra of Beautiful Soap and Co.. He uses no alcohols, animal products or petroleum products. Ingredients including olive oil, jojoba oil,

Vitamin E and other organic ingredients that they grow on their family farm.

**4) Toothpastes**

We like Tom's of Maine, because this well-known and well-respected company not only lists all ingredients on its labels, all fairly minimally changed from their natural sources, but they take the trouble to explain the purpose and source of each ingredient as well on their labels. For this decency and greatly admirable respect shown toward the consumer, we admire Tom's very much, even if Colgate-Palmolive bought them out. Jason's also has excellent toothpastes.

**5) Skin softener**

During the winter, membranes in the nostrils can get dry and cracked. To correct this, keep a teaspoon or so of olive oil in a tiny container in the bathroom. When the nostrils get dry and itchy, gently rub some olive oil inside each one.

Why is this list so short? Well, when you get down to it, there is little else that is really needed than this. Sure, shaving cream, moisturizing lotion, and other preparations are useful. In general, we have found that when these products are needed, much more benign ingredients are found in those products in health food stores rather than in supermarkets and pharmacies.

# Chapter 47
# Unconsciousness: what to do after you call 911 and while you are waiting for the ambulance

The American Journal of Emergency Medicine recently reported the use of an acupuncture point to bring a patient out of a deep coma. The report reads in part:

"Examination showed a deep coma (Glasgow Coma Scale 3) with weak muscle tone and no reaction to strong pain stimulus at the neck. . . .Even on repeated strong pain stimulus during transport to the emergency vehicle and while inserting an intravenous cannula, she did not show any further reaction. The emergency physician, an anesthetist who was also trained in acupuncture, inserted an acupuncture needle into the acupuncture point of Du 26 (in Chinese: Suigou or Jenchung), which is located at the philtrum at a distance of one third between the nose and upper lip. Immediately after the insertion and strong stimulus by turning the needle, the patient reacted with some very deep breaths and she began to weep. Subsequently, the patient woke up and was completely awake within several minutes. The results of neurological evaluation were normal."[74]

Traditional Chinese Medicine, thousands of years old, has taught that this point, Du 26, is a "rescue point" or emergency point for unconsciousness. However, we must forthwith include the standard disclaimer that any incident of unconsciousness is considered a medical emergency and must be reported immediately.

---

[74] Doyle, Brian, MD, American Journal of Emergency Medicine, Vol 23, 2005, pp.90-91.

# Chapter 48
# Aloe vera for burns and sunburns

Many aloe species exist, with some common properties among them, including their ability to withstand the hot dry summers here in Arizona with grace and strength. When the rest of the garden is wilting in the strong sun of the 5-month blistering Southwest summer, the succulent aloe plants draw on their efficiently stored water in the form of gel.

It is this gel that has made aloe so renowned as a burn remedy[75]. You may know aloe for its unparalleled and immediately soothing ability when applied on any burn. For this reason, aloe should never be too far from your kitchen. It will grow in a small pot on

[75] Heggers et al. Beneficial effects of aloe in wound healing. Phytotherapy Research. 1992. September 30: S48-S52

your windowsill or out in the garden. Too much water is not good for aloe, so if you live in a wet area, try keeping at least one potted indoors. Aloe transplants so easily and is so hardy that there are farmers markets in Latin America where the shopper may find bare-root aloe hanging upside down from the vendors' awnings for weeks or months, waiting to be adopted and placed right side up in soil.

In case of skin burn or sunburn, open an aloe leaf and smear the gel over the burn generously. It will quickly absorb and dry, and then smear on more gel until the discomfort is gone, which takes surprisingly little time.

Aloe does have a cautionary tale about it too. Pregnant women should especially take care to avoid the latex, which is the bitter yellow or white sticky substance in the aloe leaf, because large doses are so strongly laxative[76] that they can produce abortion.

Abortion is not a concern for the gel or juice of aloe that is sold in health food stores, because the gel's action is different than the latex. Aloe gel is anti-inflammatory and vulnerary or wound healing,[77] with specific action on the skin as well as the upper GI. Gastric ulcers respond well to aloe. Aloe has also been used to lower cholesterol and to treat diabetes.

---

[76] A. Koch. Investigations on the laxative effect of aloin in the human colon. Planta Medica supplement issue. 1993. 59: A689.

[77] Chithra et al. Influence of Aloe vera on the glycosaminoglycans in the matrix of healing dermal wounds in rats. J. of Ethnopharmacology. 1998. 59: 179-186.

# Chapter 49 Sunlight or sunscreens: which presents more risk?

Getting 10 to 15 minutes of sunlight on your face, hands and arms, between 8 a.m. and 3 p.m., two or three times a week, can supply all the Vitamin D you need. In fact, unlike other vitamins, Vitamin D is made best by the skin. The body actually produces Vitamin D while the sun's ultraviolet B rays hit the skin. It is technically a hormone and important precursor of the steroid hormones in the body.

Many people are deficient in Vitamin D, and it cannot be well absorbed from supplements. Even then, supplement makers usually use the cheap and useless D2, which is not the high quality D3 (1,25 cholecalciferol) that your skin makes. Vitamin D is absorbed sufficiently but not excessively from sunlight. The body efficiently eliminates any extra Vitamin D acquired from sunlight.

However, it is possible to get a toxic high dose from Vitamin D supplements.

Vitamin D not only gives us strong bones and prevents osteoporosis, multiple sclerosis, rheumatoid arthritis, Type I diabetes and cardiovascular disease, but also does a very effective job of preventing cancer, of all things. Prostate cancer[78] and breast cancer[79] several other cancers, and of all things, skin cancer[80] [81] had better outcomes with Vitamin D and sunlight exposure. Conversely, cancer patients and randomly selected hospital patients were found to have significantly lower Vitamin D levels than controls. The cancers involved were breast, prostate and colon cancers.

In fact. Dr. Edward Giovannucci, a Harvard University professor of medicine and nutrition, at his keynote lecture for the American Association for Cancer Research conference, says that Vitamin D may help prevent 30 deaths for each one caused by skin cancer.

---

[78] Ikezoe T, Gery S, Yin D, O'Kelly J, Binderup L, Lemp N, Taguchi H, Koeffler HP. CCAAT/Enhancer-Binding Protein {delta}: A Molecular Target of 1,25-Dihydroxyvitamin D3 in Androgen-Responsive Prostate Cancer LNCaP Cells. Cancer Res. 2005 Jun 1;65(11):4762-8.

[79] Lowe LC, Guy M, Mansi JL, Peckitt C, Bliss J, Wilson RG, Colston KW. Plasma 25-hydroxy vitamin D concentrations, vitamin D receptor genotype and breast cancer risk in a UK Caucasian population. Eur J Cancer. 2005 May;41(8):1164-1169. Epub 2005 Apr 14.

[80] Berwick M, Armstrong BK, Ben-Porat L, Fine J, Kricker A, Eberle C, Barnhill R. Sun exposure and mortality from melanoma. J Natl Cancer Inst. 2005 Feb 2;97(3):195-9.

[81] Holick MF. Sunlight and vitamin D for bone health and prevention of autoimmune diseases, cancers, and cardiovascular disease. Am J Clin Nutr. 2004 Dec;80(6 Suppl):1678S-88S.

Dr. Giovannucci said, "I would challenge anyone to find an area or nutrient or any factor that has such consistent anti-cancer benefits as Vitamin D. The data are really quite remarkable." As a result of Dr. Giovannucci's speech the American Cancer Society is now reviewing its own sun protection guidelines. Dr. Giovannucci's research has determined that 1500 IUs of Vitamin D per day are necessary to significantly curb cancer, by simply stifling abnormal cell growth and formation of blood vessels that feed tumors.[82]

The plot thickens when we look at sunscreens. Ingredients that are ubiquitous in the mass-marketed sunscreens, methoxycinnamate, oxybenzone, etc., have been shown to increase penetration of neurotoxins, [83] change to unstable chemical compounds[84] and stimulate growth of cancer.[85]

Wait a minute, you might think. Conventional dogma holds that sun = bad, sunscreen = good. At least that's the baa-baa baloney that we obedient sheep have been taught to bleat for many years now. Isn't it funny how every time the nastier the chemical, the

---

[82] Associated Press. Vitamin D research may have doctors prescribing sunshine. USA Today. May 21, 2005. http://www.usatoday.com/news/nation/2005-05-21-doctors-sunshine-good_x.htm.

[83] Pont AR, Charron AR, Brand RM. Active ingredients in sunscreens act as topical penetration enhancers for the herbicide 2,4-dichlorophenoxyacetic acid. Toxicol Appl Pharmacol. 2004 Mar 15;195(3):348-54.

[84] Tarras-Wahlberg N, Stenhagen G, Larko O, Rosen A, Wennberg AM, Wennerstrom O. Changes in ultraviolet absorption of sunscreens after ultraviolet irradiation. J Invest Dermatol. 1999 Oct;113(4):547-53.

[85] Schlumpf M, Cotton B, Conscience M, Haller V, Steinmann B, Lichtensteiger W. In vitro and in vivo estrogenicity of UV screens. Environ Health Perspect. 2001 Mar;109(3):239-44.

more villainous the natural alternative is made out to be? It seems like every time. And especially if no one can make money from the natural item. The sun has an especially bad habit of shining for free, the scoundrel, and thus thwarting efforts to patent, market or export it.

Check out the articles listed below for the original research showing that moderate, regular sun exposure beats cancers, including the worst kind: malignant melanoma. Also see Dr. Mercola's explanation of why sunscreens are useless against skin cancer. http://www.mercola.com/2005/feb/19/sun_skin.htm

Of course, one should not sunbathe to the point of burning, because sunburn itself damages the skin. But beware of complacency using sunscreens. The research cited shows that they create cancer more certainly than they prevent it.

# Chapter 50
# Turmeric fights skin cancer

One of the main ingredients in curry is the bright yellow herb turmeric. The compound that makes turmeric so yellow is curcumin, which has been found to fight cancer. A recent study in the U.S. found that curcumin interferes with melanoma cells. Melanoma is the deadliest form of skin cancer. Laboratory tests showed that curcumin made melanoma cells more likely to self-destruct, a process called apoptosis. Their research has been reported in the journal Cancer.[86]

---

[86] Siwak, Shishodia, et al. Curcumin induced antiproliferative and pro-apoptotic effects in melanoma cells . . . . Cancer. August 15, 2005.

Curcumin has also been found by the same team to inhibit breast to lung cancer metastases in mice.

Dr. Bharat Aggarwal from University of Texas, M.D. Anderson Cancer Center in Houston and colleagues found that curcumin suppressed two proteins that tumor cells use to keep themselves immortal. "Based on our studies, we conclude that curcumin is a potent suppressor of cell viability and inducer of apoptosis in melanoma cell lines," Aggarwal stated.

Earlier research has shown that curcumin, which is also an antioxidant, can help tumors from forming in the laboratory.

Aggarwal said that people who eat plenty of turmeric have lower rates of cancer.

Naturopathic physicians emphasize to their patients the importance of relying on whole plants and other whole foods for a synergy of nutrients and compounds that almost always make the medicinal compounds more effective and more tonic than simply taking isolated compounds. So enjoy curry in your diet. Here is one recipe that at first requires purchase of several different spices, but quickly becomes a favorite:

Eggplant curry

- 2-3 medium size eggplants
- 2 potatoes
- 2 tomatoes
- 1/4 lb (1 stick) of butter or 8T coconut oil
- 1 tsp turmeric
- 1 tsp ground mustard
- 1/2 tsp coriander
- 1/2 tsp ginger
- 1/2 tsp cinnamon

- 1 tsp sea salt
- 2-3 cloves garlic

Cube the eggplant, and bake one hour in the oven, spread out on baking sheets. Cube the potatoes. In a large pot on the stove, melt the butter and add all spices. Stir and saute the spices a few minutes until bubbly and fragrant. Add the eggplant and potatoes, and toss well until evenly coated with the spices. Then add 3 cups water and cover. Bring to a boil, then lower the heat to simmer. Stir occasionally for about 45 minutes. Remove the cover. Chop tomato and toss into curry.

This curry for all its deliciousness does seem to have an excess of nightshade family vegetables. If you are sensitive to these vegetables, you may want to try a curry of cauliflower and string beans. Use the same recipe, but no need to bake the vegetables ahead of time.

A complementary side dish to curry is raita. Although raita has many different forms, a simple one that is nice for this dish is cucumber raita. Chop up one half cucumber and add to one cup of yogurt. Season with either finely chopped mint leaves or dill weed to taste.

# Chapter 51
# Natural alternatives
# for Attention Deficit Disorder (ADD/ADHD)

One might expect a discussion of this topic to mention specific nutrients or even a time-honored Italian folk remedy or even an educational setting for ADD/ADHD children, all of which will be mentioned later in this chapter. Such treatments, as well as the standard pharmaceuticals, Ritalin and Adderall, accept the assumption that a child has a problem that needs fixing.

However, it is first necessary to turn the camera 180 degrees and take a look at the kind of mental processes and the kind of society that would perceive an active, energetic young child as an ill misfit and give him a drug that is chemically very similar to street drugs. Just like cocaine, Ritalin raises levels of dopamine, a neurotransmitter that facilitates concentration and confidence.

But Ritalin is actually in the amphetamine classification and is a stimulant like other amphetamines, having a concentration-enhancing effect on children. Ritalin is not widely considered to be addictive, but once a Ritalin prescription is begun, a child often shows even less ability to concentrate without it, and thus the dependence is established.

Numerous writers on the subject agree that Ritalin is overprescribed and that it is used to avoid having to deal with bigger questions about our culture and our values. The amount of Ritalin consumed in the U.S. has more than tripled since 1990, with young adults now using it too, and often sharing it recreationally as a party drug. As a dopamine-enhancing agent, Ritalin has to some extent replaced two other major dopamine boosters of the past now in disfavor: cocaine and nicotine.

David Nylund argues in his book *Treating Huckleberry Finn* that in our era, neither Tom Sawyer nor Huck Finn would escape a Ritalin assault on their brains, because it is we grown-ups, not boys, who have changed. In *Ritalin Nation*, the psychologist Richard DeGrandpre points to our society's addiction to speed, in the sense of video games and fast, tailgate driving and TV shows that splice together images at hundredth-of-a-second intervals as relentless forces that have helped to create both ADHD and Ritalin. Neuropsychiatrist Sydney Walker in his book *The Hyperactivity Hoax* also refers to attention disorders and Ritalin as "symptoms of modern life, rather than symptoms of modern disease." Given that fast pace of a child's home life, sending a child to a desk where he is expected to sit down and be quiet all day and passively absorb whatever his teacher's curriculum has dictated for that day's lessons is not a very realistic expectation for any child, except those eager for a break from the breathless pace of their electronic world. For a young healthy boy with no physical pathology to slow him down, such monastery-like expectations must be unbearable. I know it was difficult for me, even as a young girl, even without the testosterone jet fuel. Not surprisingly, three times the ADHD diagnoses are given to boys as to girls.

Now let's zoom the lens in on our society and our values. What is it about childish impulsiveness and particularly boyishness that makes the grown-ups cranky? Isn't it the unspoken agreement that kids can be controlled best by drugging them? Isn't it the desperate desire for those rascals who would otherwise be running through the halls raising heck to just walk nicely to their classrooms and sit down and shut up? After all if boys are just being boys and tossing each other's schoolbooks into the drinking fountains, doesn't that mar an otherwise orderly campus and belie the dignity of the academic experience?

The goal-oriented adult would probably answer yes to all these questions. But it still does not mean that our society must abandon its constitutional commitment to civil liberties and non-violence by forcing brain-altering drugs on its youth. There are other ways to approach the dilemma.

To begin, let us broaden our perspective of accomplishment and industry by looking at the quiet achievers at one end of a spectrum and the ADHD kids at the other. Isn't it a little odd actually that our very active hunter-gatherer ancestors ended up breeding such sedentary descendants that most of us can sit all day on butt-numbing chairs, grow flabby and focus for so long and so intently on the written page that just about any predatory cat could sneak up behind us and have us for lunch? Well, maybe that is a little odd, but we certainly don't need to drug people like that. All we have to do is acknowledge and accommodate their quirks with the traditional classroom.

On the other hand, the ADHD kids are not comfortable with the traditional classroom, so why try to force them into one? Great creative minds such as Maria Montessori and Rudolf Steiner have devised other ways of learning, which have wonderful effect with ADHD kids. Rudolf Steiner started the Waldorf schools, where the classroom segues into real life as seamlessly as possible. Dr. Montessori, Italy's first female medical doctor, gave up the practice of medicine in order to closely observe the learning patterns of infants and young children. She was the pioneer of the self-teaching classroom, where many different types of "work" are available around the built-in shelves of the classroom, and children take whatever work they need for as long as they need it. Teachers circulate to tutor one-on-one, or to give a brief group lesson to those children who choose to join and listen. Montessori observed that the attention span of a young child is quite flexible and ideally suited for the length of time required to learn a particular task. Children who have only been exposed to Montessori education since toddler age, and have chosen their own work that entire time end up with remarkably well-balanced academic development by the time of first grade. In other words, the skills that they have already mastered may call to them briefly now and then as review. But what really fascinates them is the task that is just a bit too difficult and that a classmate is already mastering and another already mastered and that demands their focus for a while.

And it works for older children with ADHD too. Thomas Armstong, Ph.D., and former special education teacher, author of *The Myth of the A.D.D. Child* finds that for 80% of children labelled ADD/ADHD their symptoms disappear when they are interacting one-on-one with an adult or when they are free to choose learning activities that interest them and are allowed to pace themselves. Walking into such a classroom, one is struck by the quiet, focused industry of the children and never guess that they had been labeled ADHD.

Unfortunately, Montessori and Waldorf classrooms are only becoming widespread for preschoolers, but such education has enormous benefit up through at least high school. Children finishing a Montessori elementary education are among the top performing academically of their municipalities, even on the standardized tests that are not familiar parts of their academic experiences. Librarians easily recognize Montessori elementary students in their public library. They are most often the ones asking for reference materials to write their research papers.

Just as our society is too quick to drug, it is too slow to spread the benefits of Montessori education. Still confined to mostly private schools and mostly preschoolers, Montessori-trained teachers and curricula are only now beginning to diffuse into a few public schools and to older children.

* * *

Regarding nutrients, vitamin B6 supplementation has been used with success to help neurotransmitter balance and thus performance in ADHD kids. However, also keep in mind that nutritional deficiencies can easily spring from the same culture that gave us video games, microwaves and fast-flashing TV. In our haste, we heat up overly processed food for our kids, and skimp on the truly strong calcium bearing foods: raw milk and dark leafy green vegetables. Also, remember that supplementing vitamin B6 isn't nearly as helpful as the entire B-complex, because the B vitamins work synergistically. The best way to ensure adequate B-vitamin intake is with a wide range of whole foods, and particularly the organ meats, such as liver and kidneys, where the B-vitamins are most concentrated.

Maria Montessori was not the only ADHD remedy to come out of Italy. A traditional Sicilian remedy for highly active boys who are on their way to a sedentary classroom for the day is a shot of espresso. A stimulant, but not nearly as brain altering as the amphetamines Ritalin and Adderall, coffee has the paradoxical effect of calming and focusing kids. A consequent addiction to coffee has to then be weighed against the introduction of a synthetic pharmaceutical that is almost identical in its molecular structure and biochemical effect on dopamine as cocaine.

But even more, the kind of viewpoint that marginalizes, labels and medicates the most energetic of our children should be brought into question. Bizarre as that viewpoint is, we should be able to imagine healthy solutions for it without drugging it.

Additional reading:

Thomas Armstrong, *The Myth of the A.D.D. Child*
Richard DeGrandpre, *Ritalin Nation*
Dan Kindlon and Michael Thompson, *Raising Cain*
Maria Montessori, *The Secret of Childhood.*
Maria Montessori, *The Abundant Mind*
William Pollack, *Real Boys' Voices*
Sydney Walker, *The Hyperactivity Hoax*

# Chapter 52
# Parkinsons, Alzheimers, Lou Gehrig's Disease – same cause?

Vancouver neuroscientist Dr. Chris Shaw is completing research that shows a link between Parkinsons, Alzheimers and Lou Gehrig's Disease (known also as ALS or amyotrophic lateral sclerosis). What they have in common is that they are induced, at least for many patients, by aluminum hydroxide in vaccines.

Well, we already knew that aluminum has been found in high quantity in the autopsied brains of Alzheimers victims. That's why we've been nagging our loved ones to toss out the aluminum coated pots and pans and aluminum deodorant. But now there is evidence of aluminum hydroxide in vaccines being a cause of Parkinsons and ALS also, two diseases that are considered "idiopathic" (or of unknown cause) by conventional medicine.

What is aluminum doing in vaccines?

Doctors have been injecting children and adults with aluminum hydroxide for 80 years, because in vaccines it acts as an adjuvant to stimulate an immune response. Most vaccines contain it. The more aluminum hydroxide used, the less vaccine needed, according to Dr. Anthony Fauci, Infectious Disease Chief of the National Institute of Health.[87]

For this reason, Baltimore University of Maryland researchers are now testing bird flu vaccines with aluminum hydroxide, because it is "an immune enhancer that can help the immune system to respond better," says Dr. James Campbell.[88]

Dr. Shaw's research team At the University of British Columbia and Louisiana State University injected mice with the anthrax vaccine that was used in the first Gulf War.[89] Because of the similarity between Gulf War Syndrome and ALS, the neuroscientists had a chance to isolate a possible cause. All troops were vaccinated with aluminum hydroxide, whether they were deployed to the Gulf or not. Yet vaccinated troops that did not go to the Persian Gulf developed similar symptoms in similar numbers, which led to Dr. Shaw's interest in the medical procedures and substances that all the troops were subjected to before deployment.

After they studied the mice for 20 weeks, the team found significant differences between the injected and non-injected mice. Anxiety increased by 38%. Memory deficits were 41 times greater

---

87 USA:HHS using Indonesian strain for second H5N1 influenza vaccine. http://depts.washington.edu/einet.
88 Sircus, Mark OMD. Another poison pediatricians inject in babies. http://www.mercuryexposure.info.
89 http://www.straight.com/content.cfm?id=16717

than the memory errors among non-vaccinated mice. Allergic skin reactions increased 20 percent. After sacrificing the mice, tissue samples showed that neural tissue was dying. In the mice's brains, 35% of the cells were destroying themselves.

"No one in my lab wants to get vaccinated now," Dr. Shaw said. "This totally creeped us out. We weren't out there to poke holes in vaccines. But all of a sudden, oh my God --- we've got neuron death!"

Dr. Shaw's paper concludes with a question: "Whether the risk of protection from a dreaded disease outweighs the risk of toxicity is a question that demands our urgent attention."

In the entire 80 years of aluminum hydroxide use in vaccines, Dr. Shaw's 20-week study is the first paper to examine effects on any species beyond the first few weeks.

**Do you know where to get your state's vaccine exemption forms?**

If you don't yet have the legal forms to protect your child and yourself from vaccination, look at the website of Vaccination Liberation at www.vaclib.org/legal/stateresource.htm where you will find current laws and exemptions procedures for the various states and Canada.

Please note that a few states, such as West Virginia, have very strict vaccination requirements. If you have to deal with such a state government, our recommendation is to protect your child any way that you can, including the various suggestions on the Vaclib website. If the other suggestions are not feasible, one additional recommendation of ours is to join with like-minded parents to do your own informal study of non-vaccinated children and their health, growth and development. When you are then pressured to vaccinate, inform the physician or school that your child is under contract not to receive any different vaccines from those used in the research study. (Of course, details about the research team are confidential, and on a "need to know" basis only.)

# Chapter 53
# Foggy brain syndrome

We admit we simply made up the name of this syndrome, but it seems to be common enough that it merits its own category. Many things including what you may not suspect contribute to a feeling of a constant mental block, sluggishness, forgetfulness and resulting frustration. Some of the causes are as follows:

- **Candida** is a very common cause of foggy brain. As a systemic (body-wide) pathogenic invader, candida's symptoms can involve many organ systems, including brain function.
- **Aging** In Breaking the Age Barrier, authors Wassef and Torkos claim that by age 50 blood flow to the brain has dropped by about 20 percent. Arterial plaque in the vessels that supply the brain, the carotid arteries, narrow the

diameter of these blood-giving vessels, which reduces the flow, and thus reduces the brain's best advantage for full-functioning. Thus we end up walking into a room only to find we've forgotten what we came in for, or can't think of something we recently learned.

- **Medications**: Over the counter and prescription medications have been notorious for decreasing optimum brain functioning. The same mechanisms that stop transmission of pain signals and other symptom awareness are also capable of interfering with thoughts that also transmit via neurons.
- **Alcoholism** But then brain fog is often the point of drinking, isn't it, at least at first? With continued drinking to the point of addiction the option to drink in order to place one's worries aside is less urgent than getting a drink to quench the craving. Alcohol is toxic to neurons and causes lasting as well as temporary disablement of thought, speech, coordination and judgment.
- **Heavy metal exposure**: Lead, mercury and aluminum are common toxic metals that many of us are storing in our fat cells. Since the brain is 60% fat, we keep these poisonous chemicals there, tightly bound to our fat cells. Your naturopathic physician can chelate out these metals, which brings your brain function back to levels unknown for even years.
- **Vitamin B12 deficit**: This is a common deficiency because it is absorbed in the intestines, which are not at optimal functioning in most people. Your naturopathic physician can correct this very easily with a shot of B12 and folate (the most commonly deficient nutrient), along with a repair program for your intestines. The shot takes less than a minute and hurts less than even a mosquito bite.
- **ADHD.** Attention deficit hyperactivity disorder was described by one adolescent patient as follows: "You would not want to be inside my head. You'd be like a

mouse on a highway at rush hour." ADHD is oversensitive and highly aware of distractions, and those distractions in turn interrupt every thought that could otherwise progress coherently.

- **Metabolic diseases**, including diabetes, thyroid disease or other pathologies involving the liver, kidneys or lungs. The brain is most sensitive of all organs to losses of nutrients, oxygen and blood flow, and the most vulnerable to interruptions in circulation or air flow to the lungs
- **Inflammation** from any cause that results in general nervous system inflammation can impede the flow of information processing in the brain.

## What you can do to get your brain back

- **Exercise**: The importance of exercise to overall health cannot be overemphasized. It has been pointed out that an athlete who eats junk food is better off than a couch potato who eats the healthiest possible food. (For a worst case scenario, a couch potato who eats junk food is diabetes and stroke just waiting to happen.) As vital as good food is to health, exercise is even more essential. It's pretty much a choice of move or slowly die. In a study of 18,000 women it was found that greater physical activity has been associated with less cognitive decline. That's a lot of women! It doesn't get much more persuasive than that.
- **Social interaction**: People who are socially isolated are more likely to have dementia and sooner than those who are involved in social or family interactions. Stay involved or get involved.
- **Education is for everyone**. Some people say college is wasted on the young, because too many other distractions early in life can obscure the great value that is possible to obtain from a college education. Continue learning new things throughout your life, and make yourself continue to

remember what you learned, whether through review or incorporation into your other activities. Studies have shown that people who maintained more mental activity through learning and social interaction had less incidence of Alzheimers.

- **Get what you need and take out the garbage.** Your naturopathic physician can test you for excessive amounts of brain-depleting substances, such as candida or heavy metals. There are also lab tests that they can order to determine if inflammatory processes are at work in your body. There are ways of determining if atherosclerosis is a problem that interferes with blood flow to the brain. ADHD, depression, anxiety, substance dependence, chronic fatigue and fibromyalgia can all manifest with symptoms of brain fog, and all of these are usually greatly improved by naturopathic medicine.
- **At least have a cup of tea.** One study found that the antioxidants in both green and black tea inhibit the development of Alzheimers.
- **For supplements**, fish oil or cod liver oil (now flavored with lemon which makes a spoonful much more tolerable), ginkgo, B-vitamins, and Acetyl-L-carnitine are all wonderful for brain function and can be found in health food stores.

# Chapter 54
# More proof that fish is brain food

A study done at Harvard found that in 135 mothers and their infants, the more fish the moms ate during their 2nd trimesters, the better their infants later performed on tests at 6 months of age.[90]

Another study in the Archives of Neurology found that older adults who ate fish at least once a week performed better on tests of mental acuity and memory than other elders who did not eat as much fish. The fish-eating elders also had a 10% less decline in mental acuity each year.

---

[90] Hood, Ernie. Moms and mercury: fine-tuning fish consumption during pregnancy. Environmental Health Perspectives. 113(10):A688. October 2005.

Dr. John Boockvar, assistant professor of brain surgery at Cornell University recommends eating fish twice a week. "Unless it's fish that has a lot of mercury, it's not going to harm you. And we know it improves brain functioning," he says.

Fish that are especially high in mercury are tuna, swordfish and shark, but most fish, sadly, is contaminated with mercury, PCBs and other industrial effluent. Distilled fish oil, on the other hand, has had mercury and other toxins removed.

# Chapter 55
# Some natural alternatives to Viagra

L-Arginine is an amino acid common in food that does what Viagra does, but somewhat differently. More L-arginine is needed to achieve Viagra results, but the long-term effects from arginine-rich foods are no worse than the nuts, seeds, carob and chocolate in which arginine is found.

Nitric oxide is a substance naturally occurring in the body that relaxes blood vessels enough to allow them to fill with blood. In the case of enhancing the effect of penile performance, blood flows into the penis, which causes the stiffening effect that enables male sexual performance.

Viagra allows the body to hold onto what little nitric oxide remains in a man with some atherosclerosis. L-Arginine on the other hand, is the precursor for nitric oxide in the blood vessel walls.

On the one hand, Viagra has a serious disadvantage: the risk of blindness.

On the other hand, L-arginine is as innocent as some foods. A New York University School of Medicine study found that six of the 15 men studied benefited from sexual enhancement at 1000 to 3000 grams per day of L-Arginine.[91] (The D-Arginine form of the molecule is inactive.)

Another solution is yohimbe, which is a tree that grows in West Africa. A centuries-old practice of making a tea from the inner bark of the yohimbe tree is used for enhancing male sexual function. Yohimbe enhances blood flow into the penis and inhibits venous flow away, partly because of its effect on the alpha2 adrenergic system, and partly because of the increase in acetylcholine, which is essential for all neuromuscular function.

The best-known solution however is exercise.[92] Studies have shown that erectile dysfunction is lower in men who have active physical exercise regimens. This has much to do with the cardiovascular health of men who exercise. Erectile dysfunction is primarily a blood vessel problem. And we know that blood vessel health is best protected with exercise, adequate water intake, avoidance of pesticides and other toxins, as well as regular use of a good quality distilled fish oil and/or flax oil.

---

[91] Stanislov R. Nikolova V. Treatment of erectile dysfunction with Pynogenol and L-arginine. J Sex Marital Ther. 2003 May-Jun. 29(3): 207-13.

[92] Sexual dysfunction not limited to U.S. http://www.mercola.com/2004/sep/18/chinese_men.htm

# Chapter 56
# Laughter burns calories

Vanderbilt University researchers presenting at an annual European Congress on Obesity discussed their findings regarding laughter and weight loss. Subjects were seated in front of TVs with comedy clips while researchers measured how much oxygen they inhaled versus how much oxygen they exhaled. These respiration measurements are considered to be the gold standard for determining energy burning, or calorie consumption during a given time period. They found that if you laugh 10 to 15 minutes per day, you could burn an extra 50 calories everyday, which would translate to 4.4 lbs lost in a year, due to laughing alone.[93]

[93] Reuters. Laugh out loud to burn a few calories. MSNBC. June 4, 2005. http://www.msnbc.msn.com/id/8092720.

# Chapter 57
# Happiness and good health

Heath care professionals and medical students sometimes find themselves face-to-face with an individual who feels suicidal. Many of these people have daunting life circumstances: abuse, drugs, social isolation, intractable illness. On the other hand, I have sometimes found myself in the presence of a suicidal person who has life circumstances (family and friends, physical health, economic circumstances, etc.) that are approximately similar to my own. Yet that patient in front of me has been wanting to end it all, while I feel the complete opposite. Because of the similarity of our lifestyles in other respects, I have to wonder: why? What made that crucial difference?

On further examination, I sometimes find a common thread of perfectionism, for both teens and adults who have considered taking their own lives. Needing to live up to the often unreasonable expectations of oneself or others, and not doing so is a theme that comes up. This may have to do with academic or professional achievement, or simply "needing" to be more beautiful or fashionable or athletic or wealthy or socially immersed or publicly recognized than others.

Here is a completely opposite point of view: My father once told me that even if I should one day find myself homeless on a street corner, with a cold rain pouring on me, that I should simply laugh with the joy of being alive. Just having the great luck to be the select one of possibly millions of gametes that could have become other individuals, and being a member of the luckiest species, and living on the most perfect planet in the solar system, in a temperate zone no less (not Arctic, not Sahara) is reason to take great delight in every moment of this precious life. My dad lived up to his instruction. He was able to appreciate life and good humor up to his last day of life, even though the last sixty years of his life were marred by the pain of severe injuries from a traffic accident soon after his return from WW2 service.

I have found my own truth in between these two opposites, but closer to my father's: What keeps me happy is this: Maintain a low threshold for happiness and a high threshold for negative emotions.

A low threshold for happiness means that I derive much of my happiness from everyday household events: I can lose myself in complete contentedness simply pulling weeds in my garden or transplanting seedlings. Every new flower or fruit is a source of new delight and a reason to pester the next person I see with my "garden report." But for years I did not have a garden, and for some of the year not much is happening back there. So there are other things that make life wonderful. . .

Back when my cat was alive, I derived great contentedness just from watching him sleep and listening to him purr. But after my cat died, I found other things that make life wonderful . . .

I once lived in a little town at the bottom of a mountain and taught classes at a small college at the top of the mountain. Everyday I hiked to work for about an hour, then walked-slid back home at the end of the day, including in rainy weather. The exercise, fresh air, and mountain views were fantastic regardless of the weather. But I don't live or work there anymore, so there are other things that make life wonderful . . .

I derive immense joy from my son, playing with him, teaching him, watching him grow. But for most of my life, I did not have a child, and my joy came from teaching other youth, volunteering at an emergency room and many other activities.

In other words, your source of happiness does not require special events or lots of money or unusual circumstances or particular locations or individuals. Happiness is not miles away on a distant beach or cruise ship or casino or on Mt. Everest; it lies no further than the boundaries of your house or yard or workplace or neighborhood. It consists of nothing more or less than those activities, people, or experiences that bring you the most pleasure and fulfillment and/or hope for the future.

My second rule is to maintain a high threshold for negative emotions, which can also be stated as "don't let things get you down." For example, bad drivers inspire irritability in other drivers. But I am in the habit of being grateful for all kinds of things. Appreciation is a skill that I have worked on acquiring. So when I am near a driver that would irritate others, I feel happy that all of us on the road at this time have escaped the accident that the bad driver is rushing toward.

Sad or mildly depressed patients whom I meet sometimes admit to making themselves sad in order to accompany a loved one's bad mood. Also, quite often patients have made major life decisions against their own desires but in order to please a parent or other loved one. A healthier approach is empathy for that loved one, who may be suffering from oppressive mental constraints or dragging themselves through a miserable purgatory. But you have no obligation to follow them into that purgatory. Make your major life decisions wisely and calmly and following your own best judgment, because it is you who will be most affected by them.

During the winter holidays, depression can surface more than at other times of the year. Is it the short days of the winter solstice? The pressure of the New Year milestone to have our lives be more perfect than they now are? Include in your new year resolutions challenges for self-improvement, and ways to stretch yourself beyond your present abilities and limitations. It is imperative for our mental and emotional wellbeing that ongoing education be a part of every adult's life, during all eras of our lives. Browse the catalog of a community college near you, or look into online courses in an area that you have never studied before: foreign languages, computers, art history, anthropology, scuba diving, yoga, theology, history, cinematography, marine biology.

Whatever your outlook on life, whether happy to depressed or anywhere in between, try raising your threshold for negative emotions and lowering your threshold for happiness until happiness infuses all of your daily life and overflows to others, and lifts your physical wellbeing, and negative emotions are beyond reach. This is my instruction and my wish for you, and I send it with love.

# Chapter 58
# Mind-Body Medicine:
# healing through social support

Dr. Deepak Chopra says that "the body is a battleground for the war games in our minds." Beginning about 35 years ago, physicians began to understand the mind-body connection, and noticed that strong negative emotions or thoughts, such as worry or anger or grief can manifest tangible disease in parts of the body even far-removed from the brain. This has been seen especially strongly with cancer, but has also been correlated in such diverse diseases as multiple sclerosis, heart disease and irritable bowel syndrome. Dr. James Sensenig has another way of looking at it: "Mud slides downhill." The battles taking place in our mind scatter harmful debris throughout the rest of us.

Negative emotions very often arise from or are worsened by a lack of social support. This can be as simple as the frustrated feeling that nobody appreciates or understands us, or the very practical problem of having excessive obligations without receiving the support from others that we need. Sometimes we can feel at loggerheads with those around us and must not only work to accomplish everything that we set out to do, but must also have conflicts with uncooperative or difficult people in order to get everything done.

The exact opposite of such a difficult situation is social support: putting yourself among those who best understand you, sympathize with what you want to do and are eager to help. This desirable situation is as much nourishment for the spirit as healthy food nourishes the body. Studies at Stanford University have shown that women with breast cancer who participated in a social support group had double the survival rate of the women who were not participants in such a group.[94] In fact, one of the studies was so impressive that the researchers stopped it, because it was unethical to exclude the women in the control group from the benefits of the social support group.

Many other studies have since confirmed that when people with life-threatening illnesses, including AIDS and various types of cancer, engage in social support groups, in which they offer hope to each other, the outcome from the disease is much better, usually better than drug treatment. It has been found that with heart attack patients, if a nurse or social worker calls them once a week after their discharge from the hospital, their death rate drops by 50%. No pharmaceutical accomplishes so much. If you are ill or overworked, ask for help from others. Or at least talk through difficulties with a thoughtful, sympathetic family member or friend. It may save your life and health.

---

[94] Turner-Cobb, Sephton, et al. Social support and salivary cortisol in women with metastatic breast cancer. Psychosomatic Medicine. 62:337-45. 2000.

# Chapter 59
# Who will make you well?

We have seen the triumphs as well as the limitations of allopathic medicine. On the one hand, it is to the great credit of allopathic medicine that if you suffer a stroke, car accident or other emergency, an ambulance can arrive in mere minutes and whisk you away to a nearby hospital where heroic life-saving interventions could save you from otherwise certain disability or death. The ingenious use of technology for such areas as imaging and intervention in extreme physical disability is a great hallmark of western allopathic medicine.

On the other hand, the very triumphs and strengths of allopathic medicine have given it a conceit that it cannot afford: that it would be capable of treating every kind of human illness. This is simply not so, and its efforts to treat everything, without referring outside of itself, has very ugly consequences. 55,000 people are known to have died from use of the painkiller drug Vioxx. This is over twenty times as many people who were killed on 9/11, yet all has been quickly forgotten and forgiven. Merck's stock prices took a light slap on the wrist, while business roared on briskly. Other equally dangerous drugs stay on the market, deaths from prescription drugs soar ever higher, and the FDA remains oblivious to the mass slaughter and utterly impotent as defenders of public safety. Not only that, but class action lawsuits were recently made all but impossible by the federal government, which was just in time for Merck to escape the wrath of families of Vioxx victims. Saved by crony politicians once again.

The well-informed consumer sees the good and bad of allopathic medicine for what it is and what it can offer, what it does well, and on the other hand, who it butchers and buries. Then we say, well, if they can't make me well, then who can?

Is it the naturopathic physicians, the chiropractors, the acupuncturists, the massage therapists? Yes and no. Because naturopaths treat the whole person and treat the cause, and because we are trained in four-year medical schools, with all of the allopathic medical curriculum as well as the natural treatment modalities and the approach of treating the whole person, finding the cause and prevention, naturopaths are your best bet for figuring out what is wrong, what are the consequences of not fixing it, and how to fix it with various options for treatment.

But who is it who will make you well? You. You are the necessary and sufficient condition for the result of your own improved health. You are the rate-limiting step in the chain of biochemical reactions that ultimately result in a more comfortable-feeling, fulfilled, life-enjoying person. The delusional fantasy of "give me a pill, doc, and make me better" has never been fulfilled and won't start with you.

Improved health starts with commitment: the commitment necessary to change the foods you eat to those that will nourish you and agree with your metabolic type, and to eliminate those that are just dragging you down. It also involves the commitment to exercise, and beyond that, to stretch the imagination to determine what kind of exercise or sport is fun enough for you to actually get out of your chair and go do it.

Improved health also involves recognizing self-attacking patterns of thought, emotions, behavior, relationships and lifestyle that may be causing you harm and disharmony and disruption of your wellbeing.

Who will make you well? You will. You may want to plan a complete recovery by consulting a naturopathic physician to figure out the best path forward. If so, then go for it. But ultimately, you are the catalyst for achievement of your own best possible state of health.